Contemporary Developments and Perspectives in International Health Security - Volume 3

*Edited by Stanislaw P. Stawicki,
Ricardo Izurieta, Michael S. Firstenberg
and Sagar C. Galwankar*

Published in London, United Kingdom

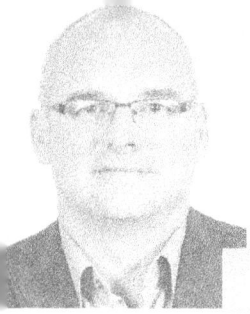
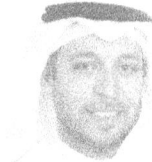
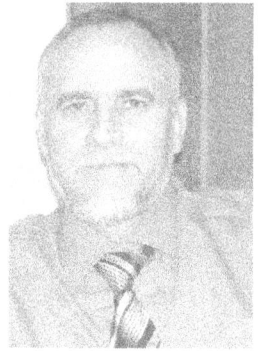
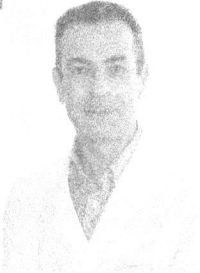
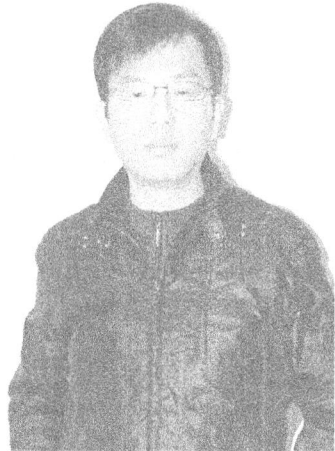
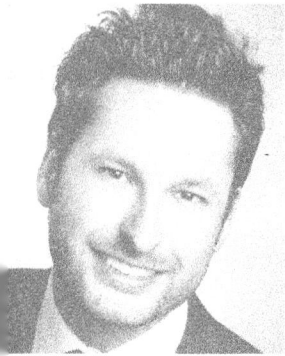
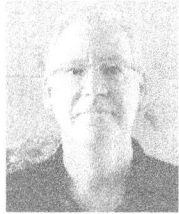

IntechOpen

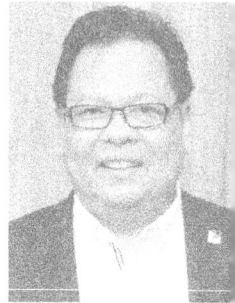
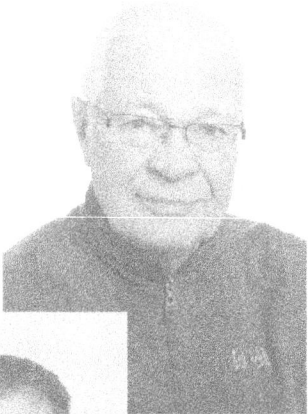
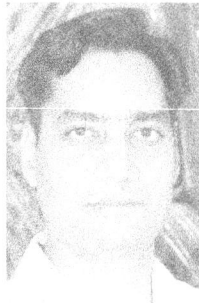
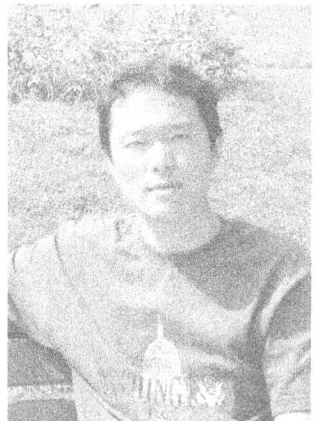
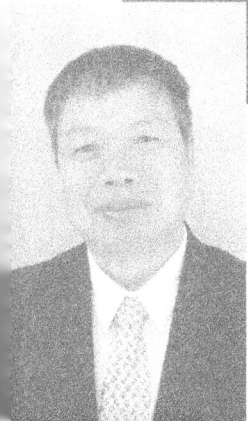
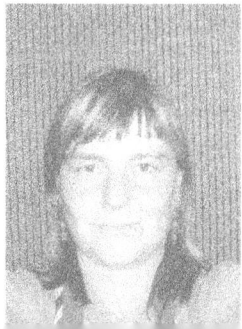

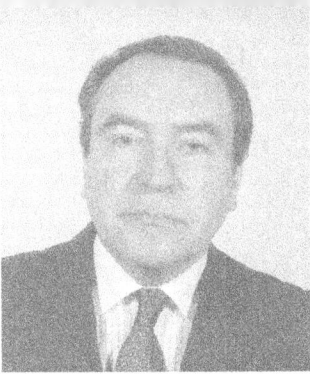

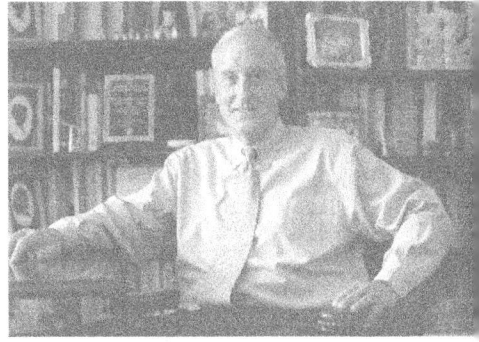

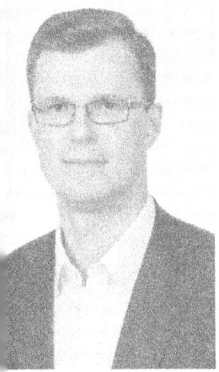

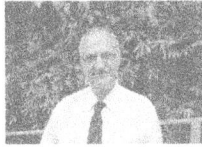

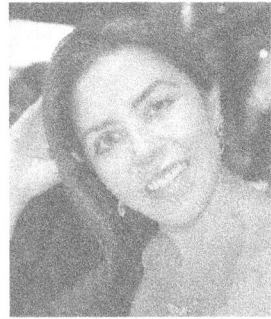

Supporting open minds since 2005

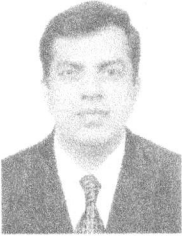

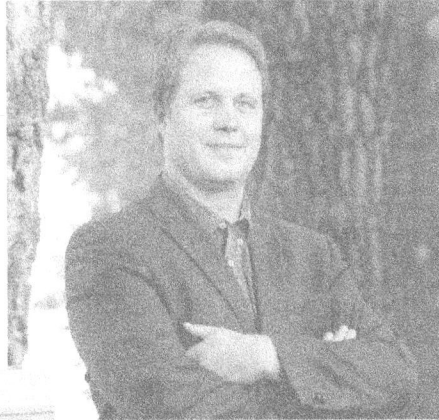

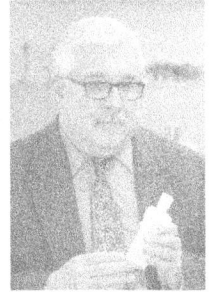

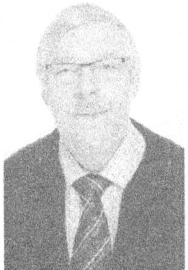

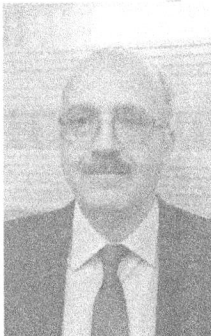

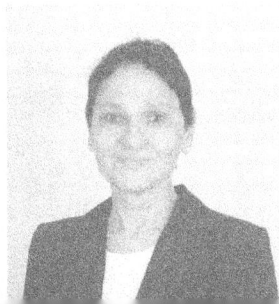

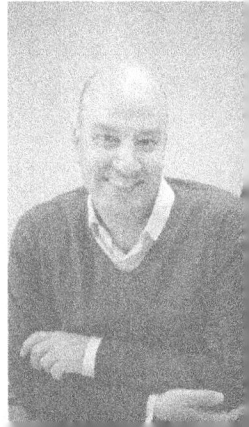

Contemporary Developments and Perspectives in International Health Security – Volume 3
http://dx.doi.org/10.5772/intechopen.97845
Edited by Stanislaw P. Stawicki, Ricardo Izurieta, Michael S. Firstenberg and Sagar C. Galwankar

Contributors
Stephen C. Morris, Divyesh Kumar, Stanislaw P. Stawicki, Vikas Yellapu, Samuel Malan, Brandon Merkert, Hetal Kharecha, Ambreen Alam, Marcelo Borges Cavalcante, Ana Nery Melo Cavalcante, Rosa Livia Freitas de Almeida, Ana Raquel Jucá Parente, Denise Nunes Oliveira, Candice Torres de Melo Bezerra Cavalcante, Jucier Gonçalves Júnior, Yuri de Sousa Cavalcante, Nicolly Castelo Branco Chaves, Jorge Lucas de Sousa Moreira, Samuel de Sá Barreto Lima, Maryana Martins de Freitas, Estelita Lima Cândido, Laura Czulada, Kevin M. Kover, Gabrielle Gracias, Kushee-Nidhi Kumar, Shanaya Desai, Kimberly Costello, Laurel Erickson-Parsons, Ricardo Izurieta, Tatiana Gardellini, Adriana Campos, Jeegan Parikh, Romano Benini, Steven Kraamwinkel, Michael S. Firstenberg, Sagar C. Galwankar

Notice
Statements and opinions expressed in the chapters are these of the individual contributors and not necessarily those of the editors or publisher. No responsibility is accepted for the accuracy of information contained in the published chapters. The publisher assumes no responsibility for any damage or injury to persons or property arising out of the use of any materials, instructions, methods or ideas contained in the book.

First published in London, United Kingdom, 2022 by IntechOpen
IntechOpen is the global imprint of INTECHOPEN LIMITED, registered in England and Wales, registration number: 11086078, 5 Princes Gate Court, London, SW7 2QJ, United Kingdom
Printed in Croatia

British Library Cataloguing-in-Publication Data
A catalogue record for this book is available from the British Library

Additional hard and PDF copies can be obtained from orders@intechopen.com

Contemporary Developments and Perspectives in International Health Security – Volume 3
Edited by Stanislaw P. Stawicki, Ricardo Izurieta, Michael S. Firstenberg and Sagar C. Galwankar
p. cm.
Print ISBN 978-1-83969-836-1
Online ISBN 978-1-83969-837-8
eBook (PDF) ISBN 978-1-83969-838-5

We are IntechOpen,
the world's leading publisher of
Open Access books
Built by scientists, for scientists

6,000+
Open access books available

148,000+
International authors and editors

185M+
Downloads

156
Countries delivered to

Our authors are among the

Top 1%
most cited scientists

12.2%
Contributors from top 500 universities

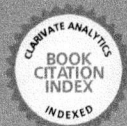

Interested in publishing with us?
Contact book.department@intechopen.com

Numbers displayed above are based on latest data collected.
For more information visit www.intechopen.com

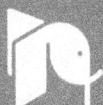

Meet the editors

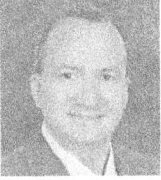

Dr. Stawicki is a Professor of Surgery and chair of the Department of Research & Innovation, St. Luke's University Health Network, Pennsylvania. A specialist in trauma, general surgery, and surgical critical care, he co-authored more than 670 scholarly works, including more than 25 books. In addition to national and international medical leadership roles, Dr. Stawicki is a member of numerous editorial boards and grant evaluation/review bodies. His areas of expertise include health security, medical innovation, blockchain technology, medical education, patient safety, academic leadership, mentorship, trauma/critical care, and sonography.

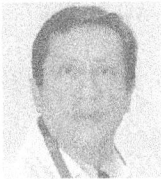

Ricardo Izurieta, MD, DrPH, MPH, is a professor and the director of global communicable diseases at the College of Public Health and director of the Public Health Scholar Concentration, Morsani College of Medicine, University of South Florida. Dr. Izurieta received his MD from the Central University of Ecuador and after graduation, carried out his postdoctoral training in public health and tropical infectious diseases at the University of Alabama at Birmingham, Emory University, Georgia, and Universidad Cayetano Heredia, Peru. In 1991, he faced the cholera epidemic that spread through Latin American countries as national director of the Cholera Control Program in the Ministry of Public Health of Ecuador. In 1997, he was appointed chief of the Department of Epidemiology and director of The Vaccine Center of the Armed Forces of Ecuador. During his studies, he has been a USAID Thomas Jefferson Fellow, a PAHO Research Fellow, an ORISE/CDC Fellow, a Gorgas Memorial Institute Fellow, and a FUNDACYT Fellow. In 2003, Dr. Izurieta was elected vice president of the Gorgas Memorial Institute of Tropical and Preventive Medicine and currently he is its Latin American liaison. He has been a panel reviewer for the National Institutes of Health (NIH), Centers for Disease Control and Prevention (CDC), and National Science Foundation (NSF), Wellcome Foundation, and served on the ACAIM Taskforce on International Health Security, consultant for the United Nations Global Water Pathogens Project as well as for the United Kingdom and the Brazilian Academies of Sciences.

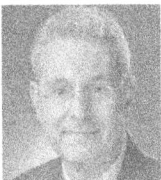

Michael S. Firstenberg, MD, FACC, FAIM, is a board-certified thoracic surgeon practicing adult cardiac surgery at The Medical Center of Aurora, Colorado, where he serves as chief of cardiothoracic and vascular surgery. He currently holds adjunct appointments in the Colleges of Medicine and Graduate Studies at Northeast Ohio Medical University and serves on the teaching faculty at Rocky Vista University, Colorado. He attended Case Western Reserve University Medical School, received his general surgery training at university hospitals in Cleveland, and completed a fellowship in thoracic surgery at Ohio State University. He also obtained advanced training in heart failure surgical therapies at the Cleveland Clinic. He is an active member of the Society of Thoracic Surgeons (STS), American Association of Thoracic Surgeons (AATS), American College of Cardiology (ACC), and American College of Academic International Medicine (ACAIM), the latter for which he is a founding fellow and current president-elect. He currently serves as chair of the American College of Cardiology Credentialing and Member Services Committee as well as an active member of several other national society committees. He is the author of more than 200 peer-reviewed manuscripts, abstracts, and book chapters. He has edited several textbooks on subjects such as medical leadership, patient safety, endocarditis, and extra-corporeal membrane oxygenation, all of which include topics that he has lectured on worldwide.

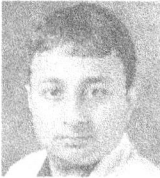

Sagar C. Galwankar, MBBS, DNB, MPH, MBA, FAAEM, FAIM, graduated from Pune University, India, as an allopathic physician in 1995. He is residency trained and board certified in internal medicine and emergency medicine in India and the United States, respectively. He has been awarded the prestigious fellowship of the Royal College of Physicians, UK, and has completed an MPH and MBA in the United States. His academic leadership over the last two decades has led to the creation of organizations and the publication of landmark scientific papers. He has received innumerable commendations, citations, and honors for his work that has impacted academic medicine globally. He has spearheaded the founding and building of internationally recognized interdisciplinary indexed journals. Dr. Galwankar is the CEO of INDUSEM, which has played a defining role in the development of academic emergency medicine in India. Additionally, he leads the World Academic Council of Emergency Medicine (WACEM) and serves as the global executive director for the American College of Academic International Medicine (ACAIM). Currently, Dr. Galwankar is the founding director for research in emergency medicine at Florida State University (FSU) and serves as a core faculty for the FSU Emergency Medicine Residency Program at Sarasota Memorial Hospital.

Contents

Preface

International Health Security: COVID-19 and Beyond...

The current coronavirus (COVID-19) pandemic has changed virtually every aspect of our existence for generations to come. It has transformed our healthcare systems and re-defined (and reinforced) our understanding of the exclamation, carpe diem. During these turbulent times, humanity came together to devise novel treatments, vaccines, and other far-reaching scientific and clinical advances. It is the editors' hope that the pandemic is now on its "last legs" and that a "new normal" will continue to be restored over the next several years.

This book reflects this out-of-pandemic transition while ensuring that our focus on overall "health security" remains laser sharp, primarily because numerous international health security threats remain. Among the biggest and most pronounced contemporary challenges is climate change. As these words are being written, forest fires rage across numerous geographic areas of the world, while a combination of unpredictable flooding and droughts (due in large part to climate-dependent redistribution of water resources) threatens to make entire regions of the planet uninhabitable. Along with climate change, we are very likely to see an increase in natural disasters and various other health risks. Among these emerging health risks are malnutrition/food insecurity, the appearance of invasive species, and acceleration in the discovery of novel pathogens. Accordingly, these "continuation and readiness" themes are incorporated into this collection of chapters.

The reader's journey begins with several important chapters on COVID-19. The editors' focus was to specifically highlight areas not previously touched upon in this book series. Topics discussed in the first section of the book include the effects of COVID-19 on pregnancy and the perinatal period, the pandemic-related appearance of toxic stress, as well as lessons learned during the pandemic. The reader's attention is then shifted to the topics of climate change and its effects on human health and wellbeing, as well as the importance of system-wide adaptation in the context of the anticipated increase in natural disaster frequency and severity. An important discussion on occupational accidents then follows. In this manner, we hope to "transition" the focus of any future work away from the COVID-19 pandemic and toward the overarching issue of climate change and its impact on humans.

In conclusion, the editors of this third volume in the International Health Security series hope that the reader will discover a valuable resource that is both comprehensive and easily accessible. When we began this book series, we did not expect that it would evolve into a multi-tome collection. We certainly hope that the continued success of the initial installments in the series, along with the addition of the current book, will provide justification for further work in this important area.

Stanislaw P. Stawicki
Department of Research and Innovation,
St. Luke's University Health Network,
Bethlehem, Pennsylvania, USA

Ricardo Izurieta
College of Public Health,
University of South Florida,
Tampa, Florida, USA

Michael S. Firstenberg
Department of Research and Special Projects,
William Novick Global Cardiac Alliance,
Memphis, Tennessee, USA

Sagar C. Galwankar
Department of Emergency Medicine,
Sarasota Memorial Hospital,
Florida State University College of Medicine,
Emergency Medicine Residency Program,
Sarasota, Florida, USA

Section 1

Introduction

Chapter 1

Introductory Chapter: Transitioning International Health Security Focus from COVID-19 Pandemic to Climate Change

Stanislaw P. Stawicki, Ricardo Izurieta,
Michael S. Firstenberg and Sagar C. Galwankar

1. Introduction

The current Coronavirus Disease 2019 (COVID-19) pandemic has changed virtually every aspect of our societal matrix and daily existence, considered from both individual and collective perspectives, for generations to come. It has transformed our healthcare systems, how we work and study (e.g., widespread implementation and acceptance of remote presence), existing supply chains, biotechnology and information technology industries, in addition to re-defining (and reinforcing) our understanding of the term, *carpe diem*. For many, work-life balance turned upside down, as home-based work became the norm. At the same time, hands-on education (e.g., nursing and medical training) became the norm for the future generation of doctors and other medical providers [1, 2]. Finally, the pandemic also made us acutely aware that we live in a global community, and how very quickly challenges that start in one area of the world can spread and become substantial global issues. A pictorial representation of keywords and themes related to the current discussion is provided in **Figure 1**.

During these turbulent times, humanity came together to devise novel treatments, vaccines, and other far-reaching scientific and clinical advances. These considerable developments will endure both as a proof of our collective achievements when working together as a civilization and as a reminder of our ability to overcome the nature's indifference and, at times, ruthless power. Although the Severe Acute Respiratory Syndrome Coronavirus 2 (SARS-CoV-2) pathogen will undoubtedly keep surprising us with new variants and mutations, the overall "advantage" may have gradually shifted toward human ingenuity and resourcefulness. Consequently, it is the Editors' hope that the pandemic is now on its "last legs" and that a "new normal" will continue to be restored over the next several years. But, we also recognize that we will continue to see spikes and surges and variants of all flavors may come and go as we all continue to learn and adapt.

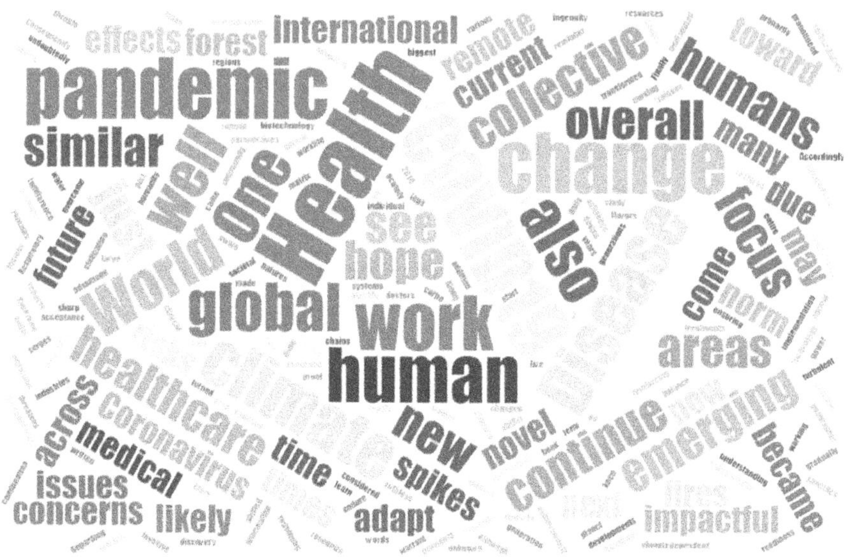

Figure 1.
Pictorial representation (word cloud) of keywords and themes related to the current discussion.

2. Re-focusing for the future

The current book reflects the current "out-of-pandemic" transition while ensuring that our focus on the overall "health security" remains laser sharp, primarily because numerous international health security threats remain. The biggest and most pro-nounced contemporary challenges are now clearly emerging, and the now undisputed climate change dominates the priority list [3]. As these words are being written, forest fires rage across numerous geographic areas of the world, while a combination of unpre-dictable flooding and droughts (due in large part to climate-dependent redistribution of water resources) threaten to make entire regions of the planet uninhabitable. Along with climate change, we are very likely to see an increase in natural disasters and various other health risks. Among these emerging health risks are malnutrition/food insecurity, the appearance of invasive species, and acceleration in discovery of novel pathogens [4]. Accordingly, these "continuation and readiness" themes warrant more attention and in-depth discussion. Regarding the specifics of climate change, what is also of substantial concern are not just the primary issues (as mentioned), but also some of the unknown and/or intended consequences that will only be fully appreciated as we col-lectively experience this global megatrend. For example, recent heat waves in England have impacted airport runway and train track usability—and hence the mobility of a work force that resulted in reports of healthcare workers being unable to travel to work in remote areas of the country. Similar concerns are occurring across the world and involve a mixed array of factors, from extreme heat waves, to rapid saltwater intrusion across coastal freshwater reservoirs, to tidal flooding and to extreme wind events such as cyclones, hurricanes, and tornadoes [5, 6].

3. The "forgotten" pandemic

When looking at the COVID-19 pandemic, including some of the more common points of scientific focus, it becomes clear that there are several topics that have not received as much attention as they arguably deserve. These relatively "neglected" areas include the effects of COVID-19 on pregnancy and the perinatal period, the pandemic-related appearance of toxic stress, as well as some of the corresponding "lessons learned" during the pandemic. Additionally, more emphasis is needed when it comes to new and emerging concerns related to topics of climate change and its effects on human, animal, and environmental health and well-being, as well as the importance of system-wide adaptation in the context of the anticipated increase in natural disaster frequency and severity. An important discussion on occupational accidents provides a excellent segway into non-pandemic topics, followed by a compendium on the impact of climate change on international health security. In this manner, we hope to "transition" the focus of our future work away from the COVID-19 pandemic and toward the overarching issue of climate change and its effects on the well-being of humans. Nevertheless, the impact of COVID-19 cannot be overstated, especially with regard to its global implications on healthcare delivery, mental health consequences, our overall collective response, as well as any other secondary implications—such as increasing reports of opportunistic pathogens, surprising pathologies and disease patterns that have resulted from "letting our guard down." This includes spikes in cancer and cardiovascular disease rates due to less-than-optimal health maintenance and follow-up availability during the pandemic.

4. Climate change and pandemics: A call to action

Climate change with its forest fires, floods and droughts, as well the colonization of pristine forests by humans is causing the depletion of wild animal reservoir species, transforming zoonotic into anthroponotic pathogens with the emergence of super plagues, a real menace to mankind. Almost all of the most impactful human plagues in history are either zoonotic or originated as zoonoses before adapting to the human host. As mentioned, it is the Editors' hope to see this COVID-19 pandemic subside; however, this is just one of those plagues that have evolved and managed to adapt to humans. As a matter of fact, there are likely many similar coming plagues, and it is just a matter of time before the next one enters our reality. One potentially impactful action we can undertake to more effectively face this treat can be the creation of an integrated human, animal, and environmental international health surveillance system that can provide early detection of emerging diseases outbreaks, nutritional vulnerabilities, and non-communicable disease patterns. Some might suggest that this falls under the domains of the World Health Organization (WHO) or even the United States (and other similar) Centers for Disease Control (CDC). However, the response should not be limited to the traditionally understood "experts" and should be much more "grassroots" in character. If we have learned anything from the events of the past few years, especially with the political agendas, concerns of "fake news," conspiracy theories, religious/cultural beliefs, distrust in the scientific methods, and the roles of industry—the one overarching take-home message is that there is clearly a lot of room for improvement in our response as rapidly evolving global concerns emerge [7–9]. Such global monitoring paradigm can help facilitate the reduction of various impacts of climate change, implementing a rational use of water and land, and preserving biodiversity. In turn, the aforesaid initiatives can translate into downstream benefits that could be expected to ameliorate the impacts of climate change on human, animal, and environmental health and well-being.

5. Synthesis and conclusion

In conclusion, the Editors of the current volume of the International Health Security series hope that the reader will discover a valuable resource that is both comprehensive and easily accessible. When we began this book series, we did not expect that it will evolve into a multi-tome collection. We certainly hope that the continued success of the initial installments in this series, along with the addition of the current book, will provide justification for further work in this important area.

Author details

Stanislaw P. Stawicki[1*], Ricardo Izurieta[2], Michael S. Firstenberg[3] and Sagar C. Galwankar[4]

1 Department of Research and Innovation, St. Luke's University Health Network, Bethlehem, Pennsylvania, USA

2 College of Public Health, Morsani College of Medicine, University of South Florida, Tampa, Florida, USA

3 Department of Research and Special Projects, William Novick Global Cardiac Alliance, Memphis, Tennessee, USA

4 Department of Emergency Medicine, Sarasota Memorial Hospital, Florida State University College of Medicine, Sarasota, Florida, USA

*Address all correspondence to: stawicki.ace@gmail.com

IntechOpen

References

[1] Chauhan V, Galwankar S, Arquilla B, Garg M, Di Somma S, El-Menyar A, et al. Novel coronavirus (COVID-19): Leveraging telemedicine to optimize care while minimizing exposures and viral transmission. Journal of Emergencies, Trauma, and Shock. 2020 Jan;**13**(1):20

[2] Stawicki SP, Jeanmonod R, Miller AC, Paladino L, Gaieski DF, Yaffee AQ, et al. The 2019-2020 novel coronavirus (severe acute respiratory syndrome coronavirus 2) pandemic: A joint american college of academic international medicine-world academic council of emergency medicine multidisciplinary COVID-19 working group consensus paper. Journal of Global Infectious Diseases. 2020;**12**(2):47

[3] Le NK, Garg M, Izurieta R, Garg SM, Papadimos TJ, Arquilla B, et al. International health security: A summative assessment by ACAIM Consensus Group. In: InContemporary Developments and Perspectives in International Health Security. Vol. 1. London: IntechOpen; 2020

[4] Sikka V, Chattu VK, Popli RK, Galwankar SC, Kelkar D, Sawicki SG, et al. The emergence of Zika virus as a global health security threat: A review and a consensus statement of the INDUSEM Joint Working Group (JWG). Journal of Global Infectious Diseases. 2016;**8**(1):3

[5] Le NK, Garg M, Izurieta R, Garg SM, Papadimos TJ, Arquilla B, et al. What's new in academic international medicine? International health security agenda–expanded and re-defined. International Journal of Academic Medicine. 2020;**6**(3):163

[6] Marchigiani R, Gordy S, Cipolla J, Adams RC, Evans DC, Stehly C, et al. Wind disasters: A comprehensive review of current management strategies. International journal of critical illness and injury science. 2013;**3**(2):130

[7] Stawicki SP, Papadimos TJ, Galwankar S, Izurieta R, Firstenberg MS. Introductory chapter: International health security expanded and re-defined. In: InContemporary Developments and Perspectives in International Health Security. Vol. 1. London: IntechOpen; 2021

[8] Stawicki SP, Firstenberg MS, Papadimos TJ. The growing role of social media in international health security: The good, the bad, and the ugly. In: InGlobal Health Security. Cham: Springer; 2020. pp. 341-357

[9] Plaza M, Paladino L, Opara IN, Firstenberg MS, Wilson B, et al. The use of distributed consensus algorithms to curtail the spread of medical misinformation. International Journal of Academic Medicine. 2019;**5**(2):93

Section 2

COVID-19

Analysis of the Factors That Influence the Clinical Outcome of Severe Acute Respiratory Syndrome Caused by SARS-CoV-2 in Pregnant Women

Yuri de Sousa Cavalcante, Nicolly Castelo Branco Chaves,
Jorge Lucas de Sousa Moreira, Samuel de Sá Barreto Lima,
Maryana Martins de Freitas, Jucier Gonçalves Júnior
and Estelita Lima Cândido

Abstract

Introduction: The new coronavirus (SARS-CoV-2) pandemic has shown to cause even more severe problems among pregnant women, increasing the incidence of complications before and after childbirth, especially cardiorespiratory problems, such as the Severe Acute Respiratory Syndrome (SARS). **Objectives**: To describe the clinical outcome of SARS caused by SARS-CoV-2 in Brazilian pregnant women and to compare the rates of morbidity and mortality from other causes in this group, stratified by the following variables: gestational age and age group. **Methodology**: Observational, analytical study based on documents whose data were collected from the 2020 Epidemiological Report No. 40 in the database of the Brazilian Department of Health, from which morbidity and mortality data were extracted to calculate the lethality rate and compare rates using a binomial test with a significance level of 0.05. **Results**: Of the total number of pregnant women hospitalized for SARS, 4,467 (46.6%) were confirmed for COVID-19 and, of these, 233 died, corresponding to a lethality rate of 5.2%. Morbidity was higher in the third trimester of pregnancy, but the disease was more severe in the second trimester (7%), being worse in women aged 40 years and older (40–49; 8.7% and 50–59; 15.3%). A significant difference was observed in the rate of cases between the COVID-19 SARS group and the group with other causes in all gestational strata and age groups. As for deaths, a significant difference was found in the rates between the first and third trimesters, and in pregnant women aged 10 to 19 years. **Conclusion**: Considering the variables under analysis, evidence shows that pregnant women at an advanced age and in the second trimester of pregnancy contribute to the lethal outcome of the disease. Other variables associated with the presence of comorbidities and quality of care for pregnant women should be considered in the model in future studies.

Keywords: SARS, COVID-19, pregnant women, lethality, complications

1. Introduction

Originating in the province of Wuhan (China) in December 2019, the coronavirus known as SARS-CoV-2 became a worldwide public concern, as warned by the World Health Organization, for its ability to cause severe respiratory tract infections. COVID-19, a disease caused by such etiologic agent, presents fever, cough, expectoration, headache, myalgia or fatigue, and diarrhea as the most common symptoms, and may progress to Severe Acute Respiratory Syndrome (SARS) [1]. This respiratory complication signals the potential of the pathogen to cause respiratory failure, the risks of which can be lethal and exacerbated by the presence of comorbidities, such as hypertension, diabetes mellitus, and cardiovascular diseases [2].

COVID-19 has already infected 122,813,796 people and caused the death of 2,709,640, according to weekly epidemiological data provided by the World Health Organization on March 20, 2021 [3]. Also, according to the 55th Epidemiological Report released by the Brazilian Department of Health, Brazil has the second highest number of accumulated cases worldwide (11,950,459), as well as the number of accumulated deaths (292,752) [4].

Pregnant women are part of this worrying scenario. They are commonly in contact with healthcare professionals and attend medical facilities, representing one of the groups most physiologically susceptible to cardiorespiratory complications, such as hypoxia, and changes in lung volume and functional capacity, especially when they show common signs and symptoms of COVID-19 that make diagnosis difficult, such as dyspnea [5].

In Brazil, a review conducted from January 1 to March 20, 2021 (from the Epidemiological Week – EW 01/2021 to 11/2021), shows that of the 353,277 cases hospitalized due to SARS, about 2,746 individuals were pregnant women, and 1,491 pregnant women (54.3%) were affected by COVID-19. The Southeast region corresponds to the Brazilian region with the highest number of pregnant women affected by SARS (1,063 cases or 38.7%), followed by the Northeast region (519 cases or 18.9%). The most representative states in these regions are São Paulo, Ceará, Minas Gerais, and Rio de Janeiro. The most affected age group was 20–29 years (40.9%), followed by pregnant women aged 30–39 years (40.2%), with the third trimester of pregnancy being the period with the highest concentration of cases [4].

Pregnant women with SARS are at risk of death mainly because of progressive respiratory failure and severe sepsis due to the physiological susceptibility to infections during pregnancy [5]. Thus, SARS evolved to death in 3.6% of the 9,500 pregnant women covered by the Special Epidemiological Report of EW 11/2021, of which 90.2% were confirmed to have been infected with COVID-19. Also, the highest number of cases was in the Southeast and North regions (36.4 and 25.8%, respectively), affecting a larger number of pregnant women aged 30–39 years, corresponding to 42.1% [4, 6].

Given the worrisome healthcare scenario described, this study aims to describe the clinical outcomes of SARS due to SARS-CoV-2 in Brazilian pregnant women and to compare the morbidity and mortality rates due to other causes in this group, stratified by the variables: gestational age and age group.

2. Methodology

This is an observational analytical study based on documents, whose data were collected in the database of the Brazilian Department of Health, precisely in the

2020 Special Epidemiological Report No. 40 (https://www.gov.br/saude/pt-br/a ssuntos/media/pdf/2020/dezembro/11/boletim_epidemiologico_covid_40-1.pdf). The proposed document has a consolidated report on the number of cases and deaths from COVID-19 in specific groups, including pregnant women affected by SARS, the object of analysis in this study. The information contained in the Report included data accumulated up to Epidemiological Week - EW 49 (11/29/2020 to 12/05/2020).

The study variables were the age group and gestational age of the pregnant women, stratified by cases and deaths in two groups: SARS caused by COVID-19 and SARS caused by other etiologic agents, such as the influenza virus, other viruses of the respiratory system, and unidentified cases. This grouping of cases caused by etiological agents is done by the Brazilian Department of Health itself. The age of the pregnant women was divided into five age groups (10–19 years, 20–29 years, 30–39 years, 40–49 years, and 50–59 years), and gestational age into four categories (first, second, third trimester, and unidentified). Cases under investigation were not included in the specified sample.

Initially, a descriptive analysis was performed to present the absolute and relative frequency of cases and deaths at the age and gestational age strata of pregnant women distributed in the two groups: SARS caused by COVID-19 and SARS caused by other etiologic agents. To learn the severity degree of the disease by the study categories (age group and gestational age), the lethality coefficient was calculated according to the following formula:

$$L(\%) = \textit{Number of deaths SARS caused by COVID19}$$
$$\frac{\textit{Number of deaths SARS caused by COVID19}}{\textit{Number of diagnosed cases of SARS caused COVID19}} \times 100. \qquad (1)$$

The rates of cases and deaths in the referred categories were compared using the binomial test at the level of 5%, with the aid of BioEstat 5.3 software. Sample 1 size, total number of confirmed SARS cases due to COVID-19, and number of successful cases in each stratum analyzed were considered. The same was employed for sample 2 with cases of SARS caused by other agents. The same procedure was carried out for deaths.

The research respected the ethical aspects of research with human beings, described in the Resolution of the National Health Council 510/16, on the guidelines and regulatory standards for research in human and social sciences. It provides for the waiver of consideration by an Ethics Committee when using data available in the public domain [7]. The ethical criteria of the Declaration of Helsinki and international standards were observed.

3. Results

Table 1 shows the number of cases and deaths of pregnant women with SARS diagnosed with COVID-19 (sample 1), as well as other causes (sample 2). In sample 1, 4,467 cases with 233 deaths were reported and in sample 2, 4,268 cases with 101 deaths. Excluding the number of pregnant women of unknown age, the stratum with the highest prevalence of cases and deaths in sample 1 was the stratum of 20–39 years (3,647 and 183, respectively), corresponding to about 82 and 78.5%, respectively. In sample 2, 3,309 cases (77.7%) and 76 deaths (75.2%) were reported in that age group, a number significantly lower than that in sample 1 (p < 0.05). However, the highest rate of deaths occurred more significantly in the stratum of 10–19 years as a result of causes other than COVID-19 (p = 0.028).

As for gestational age, the third trimester showed the highest prevalence of SARS, and the number of SARS cases due to SARS-CoV-2 was significantly higher (p < 0.0001). However, the prevalence was significantly higher in the sample of pregnant women with SARS due to other causes/etiologic agents in the first and second trimesters (**Table 2**).

Concerning deaths, **Table 2** shows that the lowest rate of deaths occurred in the first trimester, excluding when gestational age was not identified in either sample, being significantly lower in sample 2 (p = 0.0051). However, in the third trimester, it is higher in sample 1, i.e. in pregnant women with SARS due to SARS-CoV-2 (0.0147).

Data	Age group[*]	SARS by COVID-19 (4,464) – confirmed	%	SARS by other etiologic agents (4,256)	%	Binomial test (0.05)
Cases	10–19	434	9.7	687	16.1	p < 0.0001
	20–29	1863	41.7	2003	47.1	p < 0.0001
	30–39	1784	40.0	1306	30.7	p < 0.0001
	40–49	311	7.0	218	5.1	p = 0.0003
	50–59	72	1.6	42	1.0	p = 0.0101
Deaths	10–19	12	5.2	12	11.9	p = 0.0287
	20–29	77	33.0	39	38.6	p = 0.3264
	30–39	106	45.5	37	36.6	p = 0.1328
	40–49	27	11.6	6	5.9	p = 0.1121
	50–59	11	4.7	7	6.9	p = 0.4114
Total	—	233	100	101	100	—

[*]*Three cases with unidentified age group were excluded from this analysis.*
Source: Authors, 2020 [4] based on data from BRASIL (2020).

Table 1.
Absolute and relative frequencies of SARS cases and deaths in pregnant women notified in Brazil (2020), according to maternal age.

Data	Gestational age (trimesters)	SARS due to COVID-19 – confirmed	%	SARS by other etiologic agents	%	Binomial test (0.05)
Cases	1st	384	8.6	553	13.0	p < 0.0001
	2nd	1018	22.8	1208	28.3	p < 0.0001
	3rd	2784	62.3	2284	53.5	p < 0.0001
	Unidentified	281	6.3	223	5.2	p = 0.0328
Total	—	4467	100	4268	100	—
Deaths	1st	16	6.9	17	16.8	p = 0.0051
	2nd	71	30.5	32	31.7	p = 0.8258
	3rd	133	57.0	43	42.6	p = 0.0147
	Unidentified	13	5.6	9	8.9	p = 0.2596
Total	—	233	100	101	100	—

Source: Authors, 2020 [4] based on data from BRASIL (2020).

Table 2.
Absolute and relative frequencies of SARS cases and deaths in pregnant women notified in Brazil (2020), according to gestational age.

Table 3 shows the lethality rates by gestational age. The group of pregnant women with SARS caused by COVID-19 was observed to have a higher mortality rate than that of the group of pregnant women with SARS due to other causes (5.2 and 2.3%, respectively). Considering the strata, the event was more severe in the second trimester (7%) for the first group, whereas it was more significant in the first trimester (3.1%) for the second one.

Figure 1 shows the relationship between the age of pregnant women and disease lethality. The lowest rates have been observed to occur in the first stratum (10–19 years), increasing with age. In group 1 (deaths from SARS caused by COVID-19), lethality ranged from 2.8% in the 10–19 age group to 15.3% in the 50–59 age group.

Gestational age (trimesters)	Cases of SARS by COVID-19	Deaths	Lethality rate (%)	Cases of SARS by other etiologic agents	Deaths	Lethality rate (%)
1st	384	16	4.2	553	17	3.1
2nd	1018	71	7.0	1208	32	2.6
3rd	2784	133	4.8	2284	43	1.8
Unidentified	281	13	4.6	223	9	3.8
Total	**4467**	**233**	**5.2**	**4268**	**101**	**2.3**

Table 3.
Lethality in pregnant women due to SARS caused by COVID-19 and other causes, according to gestational age in Brazil (2020).

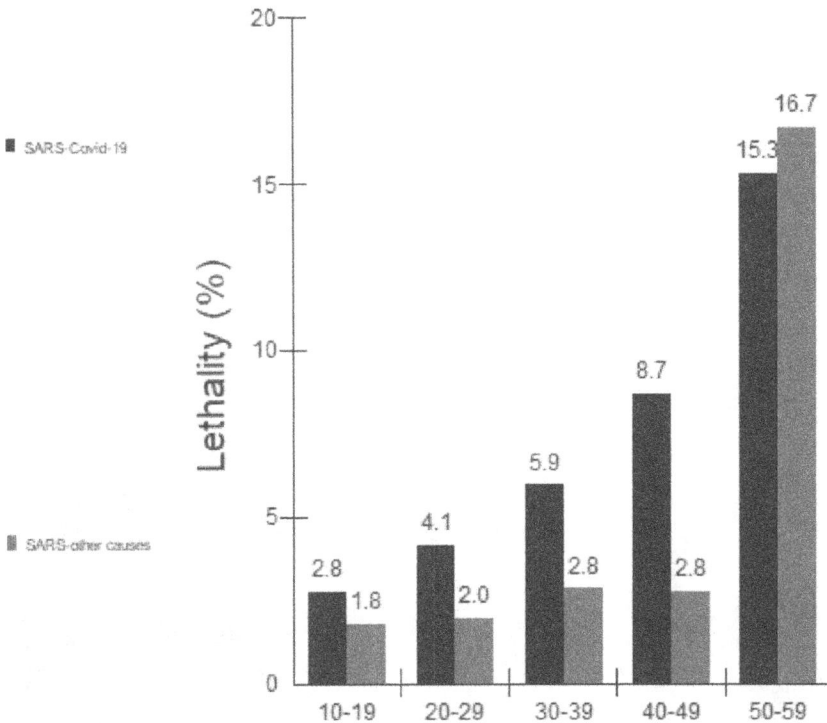

Figure 1.
Distribution of lethality rates by age in the groups of pregnant women with SARS caused by COVID-19 and SARS due to other causes (BRASIL, 2020).

In all age groups from group 2 (deaths from SARS due to other causes), the lethality rate was lower than in group 1, except for the 50–59 age group (16.7%).

4. Discussion

Susceptibility to respiratory pathogens and severe cases of pneumonia during pregnancy occur due to immunological and cardiopulmonary changes that can make pregnant women more vulnerable to hypoxia [8]. **Figure 2** summarizes the main changes in pregnancy and its susceptibility to COVID-19.

The pulmonary system of pregnant women also undergoes complex changes due to their pregnancy status. There is a compression of the diaphragm by the uterus, leading to a decrease in thoracic compliance and total lung capacity [8]. In addition, pneumonia caused by COVID-19 rapidly progresses from focal to bilateral pulmonary consolidation, predisposing these patients to hypoxemic respiratory failure [5] (**Figure 2**). Symptoms started between 5.8 and 29.9 weeks of pregnancy and between 5.7 and 30.7 weeks of hospital stay [9].

In the cardiovascular system (**Figure 2**), the pregnant woman undergoes profound physiological changes. There is a myocardial hypertrophy with enlarged cardiac chambers, which leads to an increase in cardiac output that reaches a maximum of 30–40% between the 28th and 36th week, when it stabilizes until childbirth; there is a gradual increase in heart rate that reaches its maximum peak between the 28th and 36th weeks [10]; total peripheral resistance is reduced by up to 30% from the 8th–12th week of gestation, remaining at these levels until term [11]; finally, there is an increase in central venous pressure in the lower portions of the body, especially from the second trimester onwards, due to the action of the uterine volume on the pelvic veins and inferior vena cava [12].

This overload of the cardiovascular system becomes dangerous as the pregnant woman faces the potential aggressions of COVID-19 (**Figure 2**). According to the

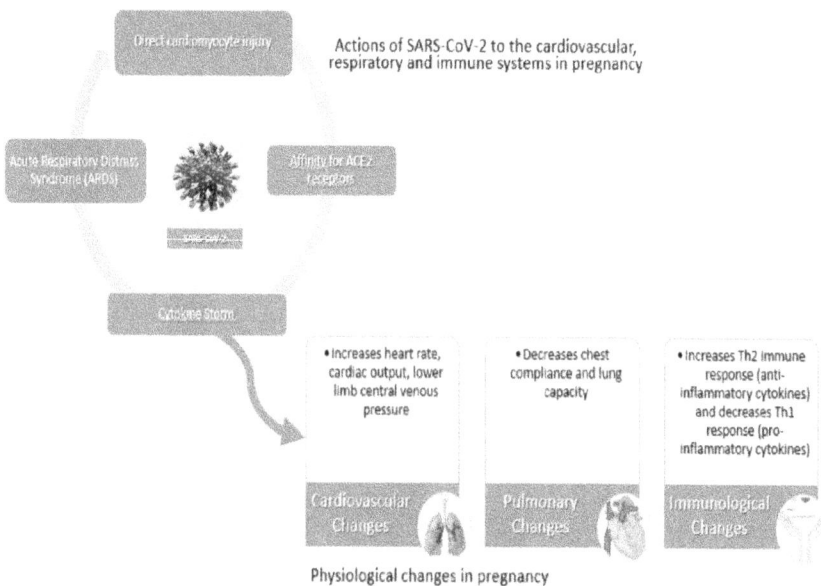

Figure 2.
Actions of SARS-CoV-2 to the cardiovascular, respiratory and immune systems and their physiological alterations in pregnancy. Source: Authors (2021).

literature, regardless of being pregnant or not, it is postulated that SARS-CoV-2 causes myocardial damage by at least three mechanisms: (I) Hyperexpression of ACE2 receptors (Angiotensin II receptor) in the cardiovascular system – it would lead to a greater affinity of the virus for the cells of the cardiac system, causing direct damage to the cells by SARS-CoV-2; (II) Myocardial damage caused by the "Cytokine Storm" – with aggression from the immune system directly to the cardiomyocyte cells; and (III) the Severe Acute Respiratory Distress syndrome (ARDS) would cause hypoxemia, leading to myocardial ischemia [13]. Thus, pregnant women, due to the physiological overload of the cardiovascular system, theoretically, would have more severe cases of COVID-19.

Additionally, in the case of pregnant women, another factor should be considered: the immunotolerance changes in the innate and adaptive systems caused by pregnancy (**Figure 2**). In the gestational immune system [14] there is a complex humoral response in signaling. What happens is an alteration in the signaling pattern, especially in CD4+ T lymphocytes. In this context, there is an important decrease in the immune response by Th1 lymphocytes and an increase in the response mediated by Th2 lymphocytes. In practice, this contributes to increased maternal susceptibility to intracellular pathogens and viral infections, which causes an increase in gestational morbidity in a broad and general way [15]. Thus, Th1 type cytokines are pro-inflammatory agents that contain interleukins (IL-1a, IL-1b, IL-6, IL-12) and interferon-gamma (IFN-g), while Th2 type cytokines are anti-inflammatory drugs agents that contain interleukins (IL-4, IL-10, IL-13) and transforming growth factor-beta (transforming growth factor β, TGF-β). Patients with SARS-CoV-2 demonstrated preferential activation of Th1 immunity, resulting in a considerable increase in pro-inflammatory cytokines for at least two weeks after the onset of the disease, which would cause severe lung damage [13].

Consistent with literature data, pregnancy with the presence of Acute Respiratory Syndrome is more associated with maternal and neonatal complications such as premature birth, intrauterine growth restriction, spontaneous abortion, orotracheal intubation, ICU admissions, disseminated intravascular coagulation and acute renal failure [16, 17]. A North American cohort that evaluated 8,207 pregnant women with 83,205 women of childbearing age (15–44 years), both groups with laboratory confirmation for SARS-CoV-2 showed a mortality rate lower than 1% (0.2% - being 16 pregnant and 208 not pregnant). The authors further report that pregnant women had higher admission rates than their controls (31.5% vs. 5.8%, respectively). In addition, pregnant women had a higher incidence of ICU admissions compared to non-pregnant women (1.5% vs. 0.9%, respectively) and also had greater need to use invasive mechanical ventilation (0.5% vs. 0.3%) [18]. A prospective cohort conducted in Mexico through the "COVID-19 National Data Registry of Mexico" compared 5,183 pregnant women with 175,905 non-pregnant women with COVID-19 confirmed by RT-PCR. According to the authors, pregnant women had higher odds ratios (OR) for deaths (1.84; 95%CI, 1.26–2.69), pneumonia (1.86; 95% CI, 1.60–2.16), and ICU admissions (1.86; 95%CI, 1.41–2.45) compared to non-pregnant women [19].

In the context of SARS-COV-2, it seems that the clinical consequences caused by COVID-19 are influenced by the patient's age and pre-existing comorbidities [20]. Sentilhes et al. observed that women had one or more known maternal characteristics associated with severe maternal morbidity, such as: age over 35 years, overweight, gestational hypertension, diabetes and preexisting asthma, which are warning aspects for monitoring and managing pregnant women infected with COVID-19 [21]. Study by Knight et al. showed that almost half (41% - 175) of pregnant women with SARS-CoV-2 admitted to UK hospitals and evaluated in their prospective cohort were at the age of 35 or over [22].

A systematic review carried out in 2021 reported that, in general, patients with non-communicable chronic diseases such as obesity, diabetes mellitus and systemic arterial hypertension have higher morbidity and mortality rates when they acquire COVID-19 compared to the general population [23]. In our study, approximately 80 and 50% of the pregnant patients were overweight or obese, respectively, before pregnancy and had associated conditions, such as systemic arterial hypertension (SAH). Obesity is considered an aggravating factor because it weakens lung function through mechanical and inflammatory pathways. In synergy with COVID-19, obesity, asthma, and mechanical stress by high uterine volume can increase the risk of premature birth [24]. Another study pointed out that 18.5% of pregnant women had at least one comorbidity before pregnancy: asthma, SAH, or obesity [21]. A cohort carried out in the United Kingdom based on the "UK Obstetric Surveillance System" showed that of the 427 pregnant women admitted to hospital units with SARS-CoV-2 infection, 69% (281) were overweight or obese and 34% (145) had other pre-existing comorbidities. Around 10% of the admitted pregnant women needed O2 support and 1% died [22]. However, it is not always possible to determine the relationship between COVID-19 complications and the comorbidities of pregnant women. In a study of 116 cases, of which nine patients (7.8%) had gestational diabetes and five (4.3%) presented hypertensive disorders, including pre-eclampsia, the authors indicated that there is not necessarily a direct relationship between comorbidities and pregnancy complications associated with COVID-19 [25].

The symptomatology of pregnant women with COVID-19 is not different from that observed in the general population. A review study summarizes in **Figure 3** the main clinical manifestations of COVID-19 in pregnant women in epidemiological studies:

	Cases	Fever	Cough	Sore throat	Diarrhea	Dyspnea
Chen et al	9	78%	44%	22%	11%	11%
Zhu et al	7	100%	42%	14%	14%	NA
Liu et al [*]	11	86%	59%	6%	6%	6%
Yu et al	7	85%	14%	NA	14%	14%
Chen et al	5	0%	0%	NA	NA	0%
Lee et al	1	Present	Present	Present	NA	NA
Liu et al	13	77%	NA	NA	NA	23%

Abbreviations: NA, Not available.

* data including three puerperal patients.

Figure 3.
Main clinical manifestations of pregnant women with COVID-19 [adapted]. Source: Castro et al. [26].

The data in **Figure 3** are compatible with subsequent studies. A meta-analysis carried out by an Italian group showed that the most common symptoms of pregnant women with SARS-CoV-2, MERS and SARS were fever (82.6%), cough (57.1%) and dyspnea (27.0%) [27]. Rasmussen et al. reported that the most common symptoms of COVID-19 are fever, cough, myalgia, headache, and diarrhea [28].

After analyzing 46 pregnant women with COVID-19 in a retrospective study, most cases were treated in outpatient settings (78.3%, 36/46) or were asymptomatic (6.5%, 3/46), with dyspnea being the main symptom. However, seven pregnant patients (15.2%) were hospitalized due to COVID-19, one of whom was admitted to the intensive care unit (ICU). The authors believe that pregnant women should be considered a high-risk population for the severe form of COVID-19, particularly in the second and third trimesters of pregnancy, especially if they are obese [24]. A cross-sectional, descriptive and quantitative study carried out in the city of Wuhan, China and published in the New England Journal of Medicine in April 2020, reports that of the pregnant women who acquired COVID-19, 55 out of 106 (52%) were nulliparous and 75 out of 118 (64%) had been infected with SARS-CoV-2 in the third trimester. The most common symptoms in 112 women were fever (75%) and cough (73%). Most (92%) had the disease in its mild form and 8% had hypoxemia and severe forms, and of these patients one required intensive care support with mechanical ventilation. Interestingly, COVID-19 was more severe among patients in the immediate postpartum period [29].

The findings by Pierce-Williams et al. pointed out that, within the sample universe analyzed, 73% of the pregnant women with severe manifestations of COVID-19 required O_2 supplementation, and 95% were intubated. Among women with the severe form of the disease, 70% developed acute respiratory distress syndrome (ARDS), 20% were placed in a prone position (in gestational ages at 26 to 31 weeks), and 20% required reintubation [9]. Systematic review conducted by Juan et al. refers to seven maternal deaths, four intrauterine fetal deaths (one with twin pregnancy) and two neonatal deaths (twin pregnancy) reported in a non-consecutive case series of nine cases with severe COVID-19. In the case reports, two maternal deaths, one neonatal death and two cases of neonatal SARS-CoV-2 infection were stated [30].

However, these findings are not unanimous in the literature. A cross-sectional, descriptive and prospective study conducted in Utah, India, which analyzed 65 pregnant women with positive RT-PCR for COVID-19, showed that 88.4% were asymptomatic [31]. An Iranian review study points out that pregnant women with comorbidities are more likely to have more severe clinical pictures of COVID-19, although it is inconclusive for the authors that COVID-19 alone can increase maternal-fetal risk [32]. A second review study published in 2021 comparing outcomes between pregnant and non-pregnant women with SARS-CoV-2, MERS (Middle East respiratory syndrome coronavirus) and SARS (Severe acute respiratory syndrome coronavirus) concluded that there is no evidence that pregnant women are more susceptible to coronavirus infection in general, or that those infected with these viruses are more likely to develop severe pneumonia. Similar to non-pregnant women, pregnant women with MERS had the highest mortality, followed by those with SARS and COVID-19 [33]. These findings are corroborated by a retrospective and multicentric cohort carried out in 2020 [34] in which it was observed that the mortality rate among pregnant women (110 patients) compared to non-pregnant women (224 patients) did not show statistically significant differences. However, pregnant women had lower saturation rates and global lymphocyte counts than their peers in a statistically significant way.

The prospective cohort study by Prabhu et al. analyzed 675 women admitted for delivery, 10.4% tested positive for COVID-19, of whom 21.4% had at least one symptom, demonstrating that there are significant outcome differences between pregnant women who tested positive and negative for SARS-CoV-2 and symptomatic and asymptomatic ones. The rate of cesarean section was 15% higher among women who were infected with the virus, in addition to demonstrating that postpartum complications, including fever and hypoxia, occurred in 12.9% of the women infected versus 4.5% of the women not infected. In that same study, placental perfusion diseases, possibly thrombi in fetal vessels, were frequent in approximately 48% of the infected women [35].

The worsening of the clinical condition of pregnant women with COVID-19 raises great concern with potential outcomes that include spontaneous abortion, premature birth, and fetal morbidity and mortality [24]. The severe consequences for the fetus result from the oxygen supply deficit caused by maternal respiratory disease, leading to hypoxemia due to the reduction of the partial pressure of oxygen [14]. The study by Allotey J et al. showed that among pregnant women and recently pregnant women with COVID-19, the chance of premature births was high compared to pregnant women who did not have the disease [36].

A meta-analysis conducted by Mascio et al., which outlined complications caused by coronavirus diseases, such as SARS, MERS, and COVID-19, in pregnant women, found that those with COVID-19 had the highest incidence of premature birth, achieving 41% against 24% for SARS. However, this group had the lowest mortality rate (7%) [27, 35]. This low fetal mortality rate was corroborated by studies such as that by Wong et al., in which SARS had a mortality rate of 25% and induced abortions in up to 57% of the whole sample [17].

Furthermore, literature shows that advanced maternal age can be considered a risk factor for the severe form of the disease during pregnancy [36]. In this scenario, pregnant women over 35 years of age affected by COVID-19 require special attention [7, 37]. According to our data, the lethality rate among pregnant women with SARS caused by COVID-19 in the 30–39 age group is 5.8%, increasing to 8.7% in the 40–49 age group, and exceeding 15% in the 50–59 age group.

4.1 Limitations

As biases in this study, those inherent in the secondary nature of the data should be highlighted. First, the underreporting of cases - only people who sought health services were notified. Consequently, mild or asymptomatic cases were not counted; secondly, the dependence on correctly filling out the notification forms; and, finally, the limited availability of information in the Brazilian Government's databases.

5. Conclusion

Comparing the lethality rate observed in pregnant women with SARS caused by COVID-19 with that caused by other etiologic agents shows the severity of SARS-CoV-2 in this group and that its potential for lethality is greater in the second trimester of pregnancy. Likewise, it indicates that the older the age group, the greater the lethality of the virus. In addition to the variables analyzed, other variables related to the presence of comorbidities and quality of care for pregnant women should be considered in the model in future studies to determine the risk level for these women and the required specialized conduct.

Author details

Yuri de Sousa Cavalcante[1], Nicolly Castelo Branco Chaves[1],
Jorge Lucas de Sousa Moreira[1], Samuel de Sá Barreto Lima[1],
Maryana Martins de Freitas[1], Jucier Gonçalves Júnior[2*] and Estelita Lima Cândido[3]

1 Faculty of Medicine, Universidade Federal do Cariri (UFCA), Barbalha, Brazil

2 Department of Internal Medicine, Division of Rheumatology, Universidade de São
Paulo (USP), São Paulo, Brazil

3 Faculty of Medicine, Post Graduate Program in Health Sciences - Universidade
Federal do Cariri (UFCA), Barbalha, Brazil

*Address all correspondence to: juciergjunior@hotmail.com

IntechOpen

References

[1] Zhai P, Ding Y, Wu X, Long J, Zhong Y, Li Y. The epidemiology, diagnosis and treatment of Covid-19. International Journal Of Antimicrobial Agents, [S.L.], 2020; 55(5):1-11 http://dx.doi.org/10.1016/j.ijantimicag.2020.105955.

[2] Al-qahtani, A.A. Severe Acute Respiratory Syndrome Coronavirus 2 (SARS-CoV-2): emergence, history, basic and clinical aspects. Saudi Journal Of Biological Sciences, 2020; 27(10): 2531-2538.

[3] World Health Organization. Weekly operational update - 14 December 2020: emergency situation updates. Emergency Situation Updates. 2020. Disponível em: https://www.who.int/publications/m/item/weekly-epide miological-update—14-december-2020. Acesso em: 14 dez. 2020.

[4] Brasil. Ministério da saúde. Boletim Epidemiológico Especial: doença pelo coronavírus Covid-19. Doença pelo Coronavírus Covid-19. 2020. Disponível em: https://www.gov.br/saude/pt-br/media/pdf/2020/dezembro/11/bole tim_epidemiologico_Covid_40-1.pdf. Acesso em: 14 dez. 2020.

[5] Dashraath P et al. Coronavirus disease 2019 (Covid-19) pandemic and pregnancy. American Journal Of Obstetrics And Gynecology, [S.L.], 2020; 222 (6): 521-531, jun. 2020. Elsevier BV. http://dx.doi.org/10.1016/j.ajog.2020.03.021.

[6] Brasil. Ministério da Saúde. Secretaria de Atenção à Saúde. Departamento de Ações Programáticas Estratégicas. Gestação de alto risco: Manual técnico. 5ª ed. Brasília: Editora do Ministério da Saúde; 2010.

[7] Brasil. Ministério da Saúde. Conselho Nacional de Saúde. Resolução no 510, de 7 de abril de 2016. Trata sobre as diretrizes e normas regulamentadoras de pesquisa em ciências humanas e sociais. Diário Oficial da União, Brasília, DF, 24 maio 2016.

[8] Hegewald MJ. Respiratory physiology in pregnancy. Clinics in Chest Medicine. 2011; 32(1):1-13. https://doi.org/10.1016/j.ccm.2010.11.001.

[9] Pierce-williams R et al. Clinical course of severe and critical coronavirus disease 2019 in hospitalized pregnancies: a united states cohort study. American Journal Of Obstetrics & Gynecology 2020;2(3): 1-12. http://dx.doi.org/10.1016/j.ajogmf.2020.100134.

[10] Reis GFF. Alterações Fisiológicas Maternas da Gravidez. Revista Brasileira de Anestesiologia. 1993; 43: 1: 3- 9.

[11] Mathias R S, Carvalho JCA. Anestesia em Obstetrícia - Curso de Atualização – SAESP, 1990.

[12] Bonica JJ. Principles and Pratice of Obstetric Analgesia and Anesthesia. Davis, Philadelphia, 1967.

[13] Marques Santos et al. Posicionamento sobre COVID-19 e Gravidez em Mulheres Cardiopatas – Departamento de Cardiologia da Mulher da Sociedade Brasileira de Cardiologia – 2020. Arquivos Brasileiros de Cardiologia. 115(5):975-986.https://doi.org/10.36660/abc.20201063.

[14] Zenclussen AC. Adaptive immune responses during pregnancy. American Journal of Reproductive Immunology. 2013 Apr; 69(4): 291-303. https://doi.org/10.1111/aji.12097.

[15] Liu H, Wang L, Zhao S, Kwak-Kim J, Mor G, Liao A. Why Are Pregnant Women Susceptible to COVID-19? An

Immunological Viewpoint. Journal of Reproductive and Immunology. 2020 Jun; 139:103122. https://doi.org/10.1016/j.jri.2020.103122.

[16] Lam CM, Wong SF, Leung TN, et al. A case-controlled study comparing clinical course and outcomes of pregnant and non-pregnant women with severe acute respiratory syndrome. BJOG: An International Journal of Obstetrics and Gynaecology 2004;111 (8):771–774. doi:10.1111/j.1471-0528.2004.00199.x.

[17] Wong SF, Chow KM, Leung TN, et al. Pregnancy and perinatal outcomes of women with severe acute respiratory syndrome. American Journal of Obstetrics and Gynecology 2004;191(1): 292–297. https://doi.org/10.1016/j.ajog.2003.11.019.

[18] Ellington S, Strid P, Tong VT, et al. Characteristics of women of reproductive age with laboratory-confirmed SARS-CoV-2 infection by pregnancy status - United States, January 22-June 7, 2020. Morbidity and Mortality Weekly Report.2020;69(25): 769–775. doi:10.15585/mmwr. mm6925a1.

[19] Martínez-Portilla et al. Pregnant women with SARS-CoV-2 infection are at higher risk of death and pneumonia: propensity score matched analysis of a nationwide prospective cohort (COV19Mx). Ultrasound in Obstetrics and Gynecology. 2021; 57(2): 224- 231. https://doi.org/10.1002/uog.23575

[20] Huntley B et al. Taxas de mortalidade materna e perinatal e transmissão vertical em gestações complicadas por síndrome respiratória aguda infecção por Coronavírus 2 (SARS-Co-V-2), Obstetrícia e Ginecologia: 2020 136 (2): 303-312. doi: 10.1097 / AOG.0000000000004010

[21] Sentilhes L et al. Coronavirus disease 2019 in pregnancy was associated with maternal morbidity and preterm birth. American Journal Of Obstetrics And Gynecology, 2020; 223 (6): 914.1-914.15. http://dx.doi.org/10.1016/j.ajog.2020.06.022.

[22] Knight M, Bunch K, Vousden N, et al. UK obstetric surveillance system SARS-CoV-2 infection in pregnancy collaborative group characteristics and outcomes of pregnant women admitted to hospital with confirmed SARS-CoV-2 infection in UK: national population based cohort study. British Medical Journal. 2020;369:m2107

[23] Gonçalves-Júnior J, Cândido EL, Oliviera GF, Rolim-Neto ML. Cardiovascular system and SARS-CoV-2 – etiology, physiopathology and clinical presentation: a systematic review. Fighting the COVID-19 Pandemic. Ed.1: IntechOpen: United Kingdom. P.1-15. 2021. DOI: http://dx.doi.org/10.5772/intechopen.97076

[24] Lokken EM et al. Clinical characteristics of 46 pregnant women with a severe acute respiratory syndrome coronavirus 2 infection in Washington State. American Journal Of Obstetrics And Gynecology, 2020; 223 (6): 911.1-911.14. http://dx.doi.org/10.1016/j.ajog.2020.05.031.

[25] Yan J et al. Coronavirus disease 2019 in pregnant women: a report based on 116 cases. American Journal Of Obstetrics And Gynecology, [S.L.], 2020; 223 (1): 111.1-111.14. http://dx.doi.org/10.1016/j.ajog.2020.04.014.

[26] Castro P et al. Covid-19 and Pregnancy: An Overview. Revista brasileira de ginecologia e obstetrícia. 2020; 42(07): 420-426. https://doi.org/10.1055/s-0040-1713408

[27] Mascio D et al. Outcome of coronavirus spectrum infections (SARS, MERS, Covid-19) during pregnancy: a systematic review and meta-analysis. American Journal Of Obstetrics &

Gynecology Mfm, 2020; 2(2): 1-37. http://dx.doi.org/10.1016/j.ajogmf. 2020.100107

[28] Rasmussen SA et al. Coronavirus Disease 2019 (COVID-19) and pregnancy: what obstetricians need to know. American Journal of Obstetrics and Gynecology. 2020; 222(5): 415–426

[29] Chen et al. Clinical Characteristics of Pregnant Women with Covid-19 in Wuhan, China. New England Journal of Medicine. https://doi.org/10.1056/NEJMc2009226

[30] Juan J, Gil MM, Rong Z, Zhang Y, Yang H, Poon LC. Effect of coronavirus disease 2019 (COVID-19) on maternal, perinatal and neonatal outcome: systematic review. Ultrasound in Obstetrics and Gynecology. 2020; 56(1): 15-27. https://doi.org/10.1002/uog.22088

[31] Agarwal N, Garg R, Singh S, Agrawal A. Coronavirus disease 2019 in pregnancy: Maternal and perinatal outcme. Journal of Education and Health Promotion. 2021; 10(1): 194. https://doi.org/ 10.4103/jehp.jehp_954_20

[32] Salem D, Katranji F, Bakdash T. COVID-19 infection in pregnant women: Review of maternal and fetal outcomes. International Journal of Ginecology and Obsteatrics. 152(3): 291-298. https://doi.org/10.1002/ijgo.13533

[33] Fan S, Yan S, Liu X, Liu P, Lei H, Wang S. Human Coronavirus Infections and Pregnancy.Matern Fetal Med. 2021 Jan; 3(1): 53–65. https://doi.org/10.1097/FM9.0000000000000071

[34] Vizheh M et al. Characteristics and outcomes of COVID-19 pneumonia in pregnancy compared with infected nonpregnant women. International Journal of Ginecology and Obsteatrics. 153(3): 462-468; 2021. https://doi.org/10.1002/ijgo.13697

[35] Prabhu M et al. Pregnancy and postpartum outcomes in a universally tested population for SARS-CoV-2 in New York City: a prospective cohort study. Bjog: An International Journal of Obstetrics & Gynaecology, 2020; 127 (12): 1548-1556.http://dx.doi.org/10.1111/1471-0528.16403.

[36] Allotey J et al. Clinical manifestations, risk factors, and maternal and perinatal outcomes of coronavirus disease 2019 in pregnancy: living systematic review and meta-analysis. BMJ (Clinical research ed.), 2020; 370, m3320. https://doi.org/10.1136/bmj.m3320

[37] Alves NCC et al. Complicações na gestação em mulheres com idade maior ou igual a 35 anos. Revista Gaúcha de Enfermagem, [S.L.], 2018; 38(4): 12-15. http://dx.doi.org/10.1590/1983-1447.2017.04.2017-0042.

Chapter 3

Perinatal COVID-19 Pandemic: Short- and Long-Term Impacts on the Health of Offspring

Ana Nery Melo Cavalcante, Ana Raquel Jucá Parente,
Rosa Lívia Freitas de Almeida, Denise Nunes Oliveira,
Candice Torres de Melo Bezerra Cavalcante
and Marcelo Borges Cavalcante

Abstract

Currently, the consequences of coronavirus disease 2019 (COVID-19) in children of mothers affected by severe acute respiratory syndrome coronavirus 2 (SARS-CoV-2) infection during pregnancy are unknown. In addition to pregnancy risks, the impact of COVID-19 on the health of these children can occur in the short, medium, and long term. Initial data reveal a low risk of vertical transmission during the third trimester of pregnancy and through breastfeeding. However, despite this low risk, cases of neonatal COVID-19 have already been reported in the literature. Historically, other viral infections during pregnancy have been associated with an increased risk of neuropsychiatric diseases in the offspring of affected pregnant women, even in the absence of fetal infection. This study aimed to review the impact of viral infections on the offspring of mothers affected in the perinatal period and discuss and determine measures for the possible consequences of COVID-19 in the offspring of pregnant women infected with SARS-CoV-2.

Keywords: COVID-19, SARS-CoV-2, vertical transmission, perinatal infection, offspring

1. Introduction

Coronavirus disease 2019 (COVID-19), caused by severe acute respiratory syndrome coronavirus 2 (SARS-CoV-2), was declared a pandemic by the World Health Organization on March 11, 2020 [1]. The infection rate caused by the virus increased exponentially in 2020 until March 13, 2021, registering 119,165,535 confirmed cases and 2,641,567 deaths [2].

Pregnant and puerperal women have been considered groups at risk of morbidity and mortality since the beginning of the COVID-19 pandemic because of the physiological and immunological changes that can increase the risk of complications in respiratory infections and the knowledge of unfavorable outcomes in pregnant women and their newborns in infections caused by other coronaviruses, SARS, Middle East respiratory syndrome, and influenza [3–6].

Some adverse outcomes of SARS-CoV-2 infection observed during pregnancy include admission to the intensive care unit (ICU) or death. However, the clinical evolution of COVID-19 in most women is not serious, resembling the general population [7, 8].

Initially, there was no evidence of vertical transmission due to COVID-19 during pregnancy [3, 5, 6]. During the pandemic, several studies concluded that there was this possibility [9, 10], with one confirmed case of vertical transmission occurrence [11]. However, all of them suggested that further studies should be conducted on the subject, as it is a recent disease and the number of participants in the published studies is small.

There is strong evidence that other viral infections cause neurological and behavioral changes in the fetus, such as the influenza virus related to schizophrenia [12]. Other viral infections, such as the Zika virus (ZIKV), can cause malformations, including microcephaly [13].

Therefore, outpatient monitoring of children exposed to the SARS-CoV-2 virus during pregnancy is vital to understand the impacts of the disease on the growth and development of these children.

A narrative review was carried out using the keywords: COVID-19, SARS-CoV-2, vertical transmission, perinatal infection and offspring. In addition to the search for other viral infections: influenza, herpes simplex, rubella, cytomegalovirus and human immunodeficiency virus (HIV). The authors searched the Pubmed, Medline, and Google Scholar databases, reviewed the available articles, and determined which articles were most relevant to the project.

2. Other viral infections during pregnancy and their consequences on the fetus and offspring

2.1 Influenza

Pregnancy is a risk factor for infection by the influenza virus. During the 1918 (Spanish flu) and 1957 (Asian flu) pandemics, mortality in pregnant women was high. During the 1918 pandemic, a 27% mortality rate was recorded, and in 1957, it corresponded to 50% of deaths in women of reproductive age [14]. In seasonal influenza periods, an increased risk of hospitalization was observed in pregnant women at any stage of pregnancy, even without associated comorbidities [15].

There were higher rates of premature births, small for gestational age newborns, and stillbirths in hospitalized pregnant women than those in outpatient treatment [16]. Regarding the occurrence of malformations in the fetuses, the possibility of its teratogenic effect with the occurrence of neural tube defects, cleft lip and palate, and congenital heart disease was evaluated. A direct effect of the virus was unlikely to be the cause of these malformations, since control of fever with antipyretics, and the use of periconceptional folic acid in pregnant women with influenza reduced the risk of these malformations in their offspring (**Table 1**) [17].

Influenza infection in the first trimester of pregnancy increased the risk of schizophrenia by seven times. There was no increased risk in the other trimesters of pregnancy, according to a nested case–control study of 64 participants who were born from 1959 to 1966 and had psychiatric disorders 30 to 38 years later [12].

A cohort study of 196,929 children conducted in California did not find an increased risk of autism spectrum disorder (ASD) in offspring of pregnant women with influenza. In addition, there was no statistically significant relationship of ASD in children whose mothers received influenza vaccination in the first trimester [18].

Viral disease	Clinical manifestation
Influenza	Premature birth, small for gestational age newborns, stillbirths, pregnant woman hospitalization, fetus malformation, schizophrenia
Rubella	Congenital rubella syndrome (CRS), abortion, stillbirth, restricted urterine growth
Herpes simplex	Triad: cutaneous, neurological and ophthalmic symptoms
CMV	Intrauterine growth restriction, hepatosplenomegaly, microcephaly, chorioretinitis, petechiae, jaundice, thrombocytopenia, anemia
HIV infection	Miscarriages, stillbirths, perinatal mortality, intrauterine growth restriction, low birth weight, chorioamnionitis
Zika virus	Intrauterine growth restriction, small for gestational age, brain malformation, microcephaly, eye and hearing abnormalities, hypospadias, cryptorchidism, micropenis
COVID-19	Intense inflammatory response and placenta hypoxia can lead to abortions, pre-eclampsia, prematurity, IUGR

Table 1.
Clinical manifestations of conceptuses resulting from the infection of pregnant women by viral disease.

2.2 Herpes simplex virus (HSV)

There are two types of herpes viruses: HSV-1 and HSV-2. The latter is predominantly sexual and the etiologic agent of 70–85% of neonatal infections. Although transplacental or upward transmembrane transmission of HSV from the mother to the fetus during pregnancy is uncommon (about 5%), the rate of perinatal transmission during labor and delivery is 80–90%. The risk of neonatal infection is higher in HSV infections that start in late pregnancy (30–50%) than in early pregnancy (1%) [19, 20].

Intrauterine infection is clinically present in the fetus as a characteristic triad of cutaneous (vesicles, erosions, and scars), neurological (intracranial calcifications, microcephaly, and meningoencephalitis), and ophthalmic symptoms (microphthalmia and chorioretinitis). The clinical manifestations of neonatal peripartum and postpartum infection are found in the skin, eyes, and/or mouth (45%) and central nervous system (CNS; 30%) or as disseminated infection (25%). Regarding mortality and neurological prognosis, mortality is higher in disseminated infection cases (approximately 30%), and a worse neurological prognosis occurs in cases with CNS involvement (50%). In the treatment of neonatal HSV, high doses of intravenous acyclovir are indicated, which improves the prognosis and reduces the occurrence of neurological sequelae and delayed child development (**Table 1**) [19, 21].

2.3 Rubella

It is an acute viral disease caused by the RNA Rubella virus of the Togaviridae family. Its clinical characteristics in healthy adults are often self-limited and include low fever, maculopapular rash, lymphadenomegaly, and oropharyngeal pain. The rates of asymptomatic cases range from 25–50% [22].

In pregnancy, maternal infections can determine a poor prognosis for the conceptus, especially when it occurs in the first trimester of pregnancy, which can result in congenital rubella syndrome (CRS), abortion, stillbirth, congenital malformations, and restricted uterine growth of the conceptus. The chances of malformation are 81% and 25% in the first and second trimesters, respectively. Rubella immunization is considered the best measure to combat this infection in the world. CRS has already been significantly eliminated in the USA; however, it cannot be said that it has been completely controlled, since outbreaks are still reported around the world [14].

Rubella virus infection findings can be found from prenatal life to later manifestations after the child's birth and development. Among them, it can cause ocular alterations (cataract, microphthalmia, glaucoma, pigmentary retinopathy, and chorioretinitis), cardiac malformations (peripheral pulmonary artery stenosis, patent duct artery, or ventricular septal defects), and CNS alterations (microcephaly). Children who survive the neonatal period may have severe developmental disabilities (e.g., visual and hearing impairments) and an increased risk of developmental delay, even autism. In the long term, congenital rubella infection may determine an increased risk of endocrinopathies, such as thyroiditis and insulin-dependent diabetes mellitus (**Table 1**) [23, 24].

2.4 Cytomegalovírus (CMV)

CMV, like other viruses in the Herpesviridae family, causes a primary infection and remains latent in the body. Primary infection is generally harmless, but it can be fatal in immunocompromised patients and cause serious fetal damage due to vertical transmission, which can occur intrauterine during childbirth through cervical and blood secretions and postnatally through breastfeeding. Thus, identifying infection in pregnant women is important [25].

In 1–4% of pregnant women, seroconversion to CMV occurs, with most women being seropositive before pregnancy, which does not prevent the infection in about 60% of babies during pregnancy. In newborns, 0.2%–2.5% are infected in utero, and most are asymptomatic (90–80%). About 10–20% of neonates have symptoms at birth, such as intrauterine growth restriction (IUGR), hepatosplenomegaly, microcephaly, chorioretinitis, petechiae, jaundice, thrombocytopenia, and anemia. Of them, 20–30% progress to death, mainly from disseminated intravascular coagulation, liver dysfunction, or bacterial infection. Even asymptomatic children at birth can present sequelae of neurological development, such as mental retardation, motor impairment, sensorineural hearing loss, or visual impairment (**Table 1**) [26, 27].

2.5 Human immunodeficiency viruses (HIV)

Vertical transmission by HIV can occur during pregnancy, childbirth, and during breastfeeding. Test implementation for HIV detection in prenatal care, antiretroviral therapy (ART) use during pregnancy and by the newborn after birth, elective cesarean delivery indication, and breastfeeding contraindication reduce the risk of HIV transmission to the baby from 40% to less than 1% in the USA [28].

Children exposed but not infected to HIV during pregnancy have a worse prognosis than those who are not since their mothers are more likely to have low CD4+ cell counts, detectable viremia, and higher morbidity. In addition, the effects on fetal development due to maternal immune dysfunction and the potential dysfunction of hereditary mitochondria in the fetus due to the exposure of women with HIV in early childhood to ART are unknown [29]. Adverse results in pregnancy associated with HIV infection can result in miscarriages, stillbirths, increased perinatal mortality, IUGR, low birth weight, and chorioamnionitis [30]. In symptomatic pregnant women, an increase in premature births has been observed (**Table 1**) [28].

2.6 Zika virus (ZIKV)

ZIKV is a flavivirus transmitted by mosquitoes, mainly by *Aedes aegypti*, and became a major human pathogen during the 2015 pandemic. Although 80% of infected cases are asymptomatic, it can cause adverse results in pregnancy, such as congenital Zika syndrome [31], which presents as microcephaly associated with other brain malformations that can result in severe mental retardation, motor impairments, and eye and hearing abnormalities. In addition, other malformations were observed, such as hypospadias, cryptorchidism, and micropenis [13]. ZIKV infection in mothers during the first trimester is more likely to affect the CNS since this period is vital for neurological development [32].

One cohort study evaluated 244 pregnant women with confirmed ZIKV infection during pregnancy and reported that 223 (91.4%) babies were born alive. Of these, 216 babies had clinical follow-up after birth, of which 130 (60%) children had blood and/or urine samples obtained for ZIKV detection using the real-time polymerase chain reaction (RT-PCR) technique. Results revealed that 13% of the children who underwent brain imaging exams had structural brain abnormalities such as microcephaly, 5.5% who underwent ophthalmological evaluation had ocular changes, and 12.1% who underwent additive evaluation had an abnormal result. In addition, 7.7% were born small for gestational age, which may be associated with IUGR. Meanwhile, 19% who underwent neurological exams had an abnormality in the first 6 months of life. Neurodevelopment assessments carried out after 1 year of age showed that 13.2% had severe developmental delay (**Table 1**) [33].

3. What we know about COVID-19 during pregnancy and the prognosis of the fetus and offspring

At the beginning of the pandemic, the clinical manifestations of COVID-19 in pregnant women and babies were unknown. Some studies concluded that the evolution of SARS-CoV-2 infection in pregnant and nonpregnant women was similar [6, 34]. A case–control study compared the clinical evolution of COVID-19 between pregnant women with and without COVID-19 and observed that pregnant women with mild symptoms of COVID-19 have a similar evolution to those without the disease. However, pregnant patients with severe or critical illness have worse results. The risk factors for a worse maternal and neonatal outcome include black and Hispanic race, advanced maternal age, obesity, comorbidities (diabetes mellitus and chronic hypertension), and admission to the COVID-19-related antepartum [35].

Immune responses in pregnancy induce that pregnancy is a risk factor for SARS-CoV-2 infection. In both normal and COVID-19-infected pregnancies, maternal immune responses occur as a result of decreased lymphocytes, inhibitory natural killer cell receptor activation such as NKG2A, and increased inflammatory cytokines (interferon-ɣ, interleukin (IL)-2, IL-6, IL-7, IL-10, and tumor necrosis factor-α) [36, 37]. In addition, the angiotensin-converting enzyme 2 is the receptor for SARS-CoV-2 and is widely expressed in the female reproductive system (ovary, uterus, vagina, and placenta) and fetal tissues; therefore, vertical transmission of COVID-19 is possible [38, 39].

The fetuses of mothers infected with SARS-CoV-2 may be exposed to an intense inflammatory response, which can induce placental or fetal damage. Nonspecific anatomopathological changes were observed in SARS-CoV-2 infected placentas, and the most common finding was poor placental perfusion on the maternal side due to maternal hypoxia secondary to severe pulmonary infection by COVID-19.

Both maternal immune response and poor placental perfusion can result in abortions, pre-eclampsia, prematurity, and IUGR [37, 40].

A study that evaluated the fetal inflammatory response in newborns of mothers infected with COVID-19 in the third trimester observed an increase in IL-6 in the fetuses, which may determine adverse sequelae of neurological development, including autism, psychosis, and long-term sensorineural deficits. However, longitudinal studies are needed to validate these associations (**Table 1**) [37, 41].

Only one study confirmed the vertical intrauterine transmission. In the case report described by Vivanti et al., the pregnant woman was in her last trimester of pregnancy (35 weeks) when she developed symptoms and was diagnosed with COVID-19. Cesarean delivery was indicated because of fetal distress. The conceptus was resuscitated at birth and transferred in invasive mechanical ventilation to the ICU. The virus was investigated and detected by RT-PCR from the amniotic fluid, placental tissue, bronchoalveolar lavage fluid, blood, and nasopharyngeal and anal swabs. The conceptus evolved with neurological manifestations similar to those described in adult patients with COVID-19 [11].

A review study evaluated 108 pregnant women confirmed with COVID-19 and found that 86 had pregnancy resolution. Of the newborns, 75 were tested for SARS-CoV-2 using RT-PCR, and only one was positive (1.3%). The test was collected at 36 h of life. The patient presented a good clinical evolution with reports of lymphopenia and increased liver enzymes in laboratory tests. The average gestational age of the 86 pregnancies evaluated was 36 weeks and 1 day. One baby died at birth (1.1%), and one pregnancy resulted in intrauterine death (1.1%). In both cases, the mothers had severe COVID-19. Seven babies (8.1%) required admission to the neonatal ICU [42].

A study of nine case series and two case reports evaluated 65 mothers confirmed for COVID-19 and 57 newborns. The report revealed that 31% of cases had fetal distress, and 38% of pregnant women had a premature birth. Neonatal complications were breathing difficulties or pneumonia (18%), low birth weight (13%), skin rash (3%), disseminated intravascular coagulation (3%), asphyxia (2%), and perinatal death (3%). Twenty-seven newborns underwent RT-PCR for SARS-CoV-2 by nasopharyngeal swab. Of them, four were positive: one newborn was healthy, and three had pneumonia and positive results on nasopharynx and anal swabs on days 2 and 4 of life. The question remains whether some of the maternal and neonatal complications reported are due to the virus and not iatrogenic, for example, the indication for cesarean delivery determining premature birth [43].

The infection by the SARS-CoV-2 virus presents neurological manifestations, which can be a consequence of cardiorespiratory failure and metabolic abnormalities triggered by the infection, direct invasion of the virus, or an autoimmune response to the virus. Among the neurological symptoms observed were headache, ageusia, anosmia, dizziness, myalgia/myositis, and stroke [44, 45]. The effects of this neurotropism of the virus should be investigated in children, especially in newborns whose mothers were infected during pregnancy, since its consequences on children's neurological development are unknown. In addition, the effects of infection according to the trimester of pregnancy are unknown, leaving doubt about the prognosis of children of mothers infected in the first trimester, in relation to other periods of pregnancy (**Table 2**).

International Health Security, also called "global health security" or "public health security", has as its main objective to maintain humanity's well-being through prevention. Its focus is not only on diseases (infectious, chronic), it also encompasses social determinants of health, bioterrorism, climate change, cybersecurity in health and other situations.

COVID-19 study	Neonate clinical manifestation
Wong YP, Khong TY, Tan GC, 2021	Poor placenta perfusion: abortions, pre-eclampsia, prematurity and IUGR
Cavalcante M, Cavalcante C, Sarno M, Barini R, Kwak-kim J, 2021	
Wong YP, Khong TY, Tan GC, 2021	Increase in IL-6: autism, psychosis and long-term sensorineural deficits
Liu P, Zheng J, Yang P, Wang X, Wei C, Zhang S, et al., 2020	
Vivanti AJ, Vauloup-Fellous C, Prevot S, Zupan V, Suffee C, Do Cao J, et al., 2020	Conceptus evolved with neurological manifestations similar to those described in adults patients with COVID-19
Zaigham M, Andersson O, 2020	Outcome of death at birth and intrauterine death of fetuses from mothers confirmed for COVID-19
Zimmermann P, Curtis N, 2020	Fetal distress, premature birth, breathing difficulties, pneumonia, low birth weight, skin rash, disseminated intravascular coagulation, asphyxia and perinatal death

Table 2.
Studies that evaluated the clinical manifestations in newborns born to mothers confirmed with COVID-19.

COVID-19 is a threat to international health security, as it has repercussions in all aspects of human health, physical, social and mental well-being, as the disease causes death, sequelae, compromised mental health and social of individuals.

In children, in addition to the impact of the absence of face-to-face classes in schools and social interaction, the impact of intrauterine SARS-CoV-2 infection on their neurological and body development is still uncertain. Being an item of extreme importance to International Health Security.

4. Conclusion

It is vital to monitor the growth and proper development of children exposed to COVID-19 during pregnancy since whether or not vertical transmission occurs is still uncertain, and if confirmed, fetal prognosis should be improved through diagnosis to determine early consequences. Several viral infections during pregnancy can compromise the health of the fetuses in the short, medium, and long term.

Conflict of interest

The authors declare no conflict of interest.

Author details

Ana Nery Melo Cavalcante[1], Ana Raquel Jucá Parente[2],
Rosa Lívia Freitas de Almeida[1], Denise Nunes Oliveira[2],
Candice Torres de Melo Bezerra Cavalcante[2] and Marcelo Borges Cavalcante[3,4*]

1 Public Health Postgraduate Program, University of Fortaleza (UNIFOR),
Fortaleza, Ceará, Brazil

2 Medical Course, University of Fortaleza (UNIFOR), Fortaleza, Ceará, Brazil

3 Postgraduate Program in Medical Sciences, University of Fortaleza (UNIFOR),
Fortaleza, Ceará, Brazil

4 CONCEPTUS – Reproductive Medicine, Fortaleza, Ceará, Brazil

*Address all correspondence to: marcelocavalcante.med@gmail.com

IntechOpen

References

[1] Zhu N, Zhang D, Wang W, Li X, Yang B, Song J, et al. A Novel Coronavirus from Patients with Pneumonia in China, 2019. N Engl J Med. 2020; 382(8):727-33. DOI: 10.1056/NEJMoa2001017

[2] Johns Hopkins University & Medicine [Internet]. 2021. Available from: https://coronavirus.jhu.edu/. 2021.

[3] Fan C, Lei D, Fang C, Li C, Wang M, Liu Y, et al. Perinatal Transmission of COVID-19 Associated SARS-CoV-2: Should We Worry? Clin Infect Dis. 2020;72(5): 862-4. DOI: 10.1093/cid/ciaa226

[4] Molteni E, Astley CM, Ma W, Sudre CH, Magee LA, Murray B, et al. SARS-CoV-2 (COVID-19) infection in pregnant women: characterization of symptoms and syndromes predictive of disease and severity through real-time, remote participatory epidemiology. medRxiv. 2020. DOI: 10.1101/2020.08.17.20161760

[5] Chen H, Guo J, Wang C, Luo F, Yu X, Zhang W, et al. Clinical characteristics and intrauterine vertical transmission potential of COVID-19 infection in nine pregnant women: a retrospective review of medical records. Lancet. 2020;395 (10226):809-15. DOI: 10.1016/S0140-6736(20)30360-3

[6] Schwartz DA. An analysis of 38 pregnant women with COVID-19, their newborn infants, and maternal-fetal transmission of SARS-CoV-2: Maternal coronavirus infections and pregnancy outcomes. Arch Pathol Lab Med. 2020;144(7):799-805. DOI: DOI: 10.5858/arpa.2020-0901-SA

[7] Toro F Di, Gjoka M, Lorenzo G Di, Santo D De, Seta F De, Maso G, et al. Impact of COVID-19 on maternal and neonatal outcomes: a systematic review and meta-analysis. Clin Microbiol Infect [Internet]. 2020;27(2021):36-46. DOI: 10.1016/j.cmi.2020.10.007

[8] Breslin N, Baptiste C, Gyamfi-Bannerma C, Miller R, Martinez R, Bernstein K, et al. Coronavirus disease 2019 infection among asymptomatic and symptomatic pregnant women: two weeks of confirmed presentations to an affiliated pair of New York City hospitals. Am J Obs Gynecol MFM. 2020;2(2):1-7. DOI: 10.1016/j.ajogmf.2020.100118

[9] Knight M, Bunch K, Vousden N, Morris E, Simpson N, Gale C, et al. Characteristics and outcomes of pregnant women admitted to hospital with confirmed SARS-CoV-2 infection in UK: national population based cohort study. BMJ. 2020;369:1-7. DOI: 10.1136/bmj.m2107

[10] Penfield CA, Brubaker SG, Limaye MA, Lighter J, Ratner AJ, Thomas KM, et al. Detection of severe acute respiratory syndrome coronavirus 2 in placental and fetal membrane samples. Am J Obstet Gynecol MFM. 2020;2(3):1-2. DOI: 10.1016/j.ajogmf.2020.100133

[11] Vivanti AJ, Vauloup-Fellous C, Prevot S, Zupan V, Suffee C, Do Cao J, et al. Transplacental transmission of SARS-CoV-2 infection. Nat Commun. 2020;11(1):1-7. DOI: 10.1038/s41467-020-17436-6

[12] Brown AS, Begg MD, Gravenstein S, Schaefer CA, Wyatt RJ, Bresnahan M, et al. Serologic evidence of prenatal influenza in the etiology of schizophrenia. Arch Gen psychiatry. 2004;61(8):774-80. DOI: 10.1001/archpsyc.61.8.774

[13] Vouga M, Baud D. Imaging of congenital Zika virus infection: the route to identification of prognostic

factors. Prenat Diagn. 2016;36(9):799-811. DOI: 10.1002/pd.4880

[14] Silasi M, Cardenas I, Kwon JY, Racicot K, Aldo P, Mor G. Viral Infections During Pregnancy. Am J Reprod Immunol. 2015;73(3):199-213. DOI: 10.1111/aji.12355

[15] Dodds L, McNeil SA, Fell D, Allen VM, Coombs A, Scott J, et al. Impact of influenza exposure on rates of hospital admissions and physician visits because of respiratory illness among pregnant women. CMAJ. 2007;176(4): 463-8. DOI: 10.1503/cmaj.061435

[16] Meijer WJ, Van Noortwijk AGA Bruinse HW, Wen-sing AMJ. Influenza virus infection in pregnancy: a review. Acta Obstet Gynecol Scand. 2015;94: 797-819. DOI: 10.1111/aogs.12680

[17] Acs N, Bánhidy F, Pu E, Czeizel AE. Maternal influenza during pregnancy and risk of congenital abnormalities in offspring. Birth Defects Res A Clin Mol Teratol. 2005;73(12):989-96. DOI: 10.1002/bdra.20195

[18] Zerbo O, Qian Y, Yoshida C, Fireman B, Klein NP, Croen LA. Association between influenza infection and vaccination during pregnancy and risk of autism spectrum disorder. JAMAPediatrics. 2017;171(1):1-7. DOI: 10.1001/jamapediatrics.2016.3609

[19] Bhatta AK, Keyal U, Liu Y, Gellen E. Vertical transmission of herpes simplex virus: an update. J der Dtsch Dermatologischen Gesellschaft. 2018;16(6):685-92. DOI: 10.1111/ddg.13529

[20] Straface G, Selmin A, Zanardo V, Santis M De, Ercoli A, Scambia G. Herpes simplex virus infection in pregnancy. Infect Dis Obstet Gynecol. 2012;2012:1-6. DOI: 10.1155/2012/385697

[21] Anzivino E, Fioriti D, Mischitelli M, Bellizzi A, Barucca V, Chiarini F, et al.

Herpes simplex virus infection in pregnancy and in neonate: status of art of epidemiology, diagnosis, therapy and prevention. Virol J. 2009;6(11):1-11. DOI: 10.1186/1743-422X-6-40

[22] Silasi M, Cardenas I, Ricicot K, Kwon JY, Aldo P, Mor G. Viral infections during pregnancy. American journal reproductive imunology. 2015;73(3): 199-213. DOI: 10.1111/aji.12355

[23] Society of Obstetricians and Gynaecologists of Canada (SOGC). SOGC Clinical practice guideline. J Obstet Gynaecol Can. 2018;40(12): 1646–1656. DOI: 10.1016/j.jogc.2018.07.003.

[24] Lambert N, Strebel P, Orenstein W, Icenogle J, Gregory A, Vaccine C, et al. Rubella. Lancet. 2015;385(9984):2297-307. DOI: 10.1016/S0140-6736(14)60539-0

[25] Naddeo F, Castilho A, Granato C. Cytomegalovirus infection in pregnancy. J Bras Patol Med Lab. 2015; 51(5):310-314. DOI: 10.5935/1676-2444.20150050

[26] Ornoy A, Diav-citrin O. Fetal effects of primary and secondary cytomegalovirus infection in pregnancy. Reprod toxiclogy. 2006;21(4):399-409. DOI: 10.1016/j.reprotox.2005.02.002

[27] Bonalumi S, Trapanese A, Santamaria A, Emidio LD, Mobili L, Bonalumi S, et al. Cytomegalovirus infection in pregnancy: review of the literature. J Prenat Med. 2011;5(1):1-8.

[28] Altfeld M, Bunders MJ. Impact of maternal HIV-1 infection on the feto-maternal crosstalk and consequences for prenancy outcome and infant health. Springer-Verlag Berlin Heidelberg. 2016; 38(6): 727-738. DOI: 10.1007/s00281-016-0578-9

[29] Byrne L, Sconza R, Foster C, Tookey PA, Cortina-borja M, Thorne C,

et al. Pregnancy incidence and outcomes in women with perinatal HIV infection. AIDS. 2021;31(12):1745-54. DOI:10. 1097/QAD.0000000000001552

[30] Chilaka V, Konje J. HIV in pregnancy – an update. European Journal of Obstretrics and Gynecology and Reproductive Biology. 2020; 256:484-491. DOI: 10.1016/j. ejogrb.2020.11.034.

[31] Comeau G, Zinna RA, Scott T, Ernst K, Walker K, Carri Y, et al. Vertical Transmission of Zika Virus in *Aedes aegypti* produces potentially infectious progeny. Am J Trop Med Hyg. 2020;103(2):876-83. DOI: 10.4269/ ajtmh.19-0698

[32] Faizan I, Naqvi IH. Zika Virus-induced microcephaly and its possible molecular mechanism. Intervirology. 2017;59(3):152-8. DOI: 10.1159/ 000452950

[33] Brasil P, Vasconcelos Z, Kerin T, Gabaglia CR, Ribeiro IP, Bonaldo MC, et al. Zika virus vertical transmission in children with confirmed antenatal exposure. Nat Commun [Internet]. 2020;11(1):1-8. DOI: DOI: 10.1038/ s41467-020-17331-0

[34] Yu N, Li W, Kang Q, Xiong Z, Wang S, Lin X, et al. Clinical features and obstetric and neonatal outcomes of pregnant patients with COVID-19 in Wuhan, China: a retrospective, single-centre, descriptive study. Lancet. 2020;20(5):559-64. DOI: 10.1016/ S1473-3099(20)30176-6

[35] Brandt JS, Jennifer H, Reddy A, Schuster M, Patrick H, Rosen T, et al. Epidemiology of coronavirus disease 2019 in pregnancy: risk factors and associations with adverse maternal and neonatal outcomes. Am J Obstet Gynecol. 2020;1-9. DOI: 10.1016/j. ajog.2020.09.043

[36] Phoswa WN, Khaliq OP. Is pregnancy a risk factor of COVID-19?

Eur J Obs Gynecol Reprod Biol. 2020;252:605-9. DOI: 10.1016/j. ejogrb.2020.06.058

[37] Wong YP, Khong TY, Tan GC. The effects of COVID-19 on placenta and pregnancy: What do we know so far? Diagnostics. 2021;11(1):1-13. DOI: 10.3390/diagnostics11010094

[38] Jing Y, Run-Qian L, Hao-Ran W, Hao-Ran C, Ya-Bin L, Yang G, et al. Potential influence of COVID-19/ACE2 on the female reproductive system. Mol Hum Reprod. 2020;26(6):367-73. DOI: 10.1093/molehr/gaaa030

[39] Li M, Chen L, Zhang J, Xiong C, Li X. The SARS-CoV-2 receptor ACE2 expression of maternal-fetal interface and fetal organs by single-cell transcriptome study. PLoS One [Internet]. 2020;15(4):1-12. DOI: 10.1371/journal.pone.0230295

[40] Cavalcante M, Cavalcante C, Sarno M, Barini R, Kwak-kim J. Maternal immune responses and obstetrical outcomes of pregnant women with COVID-19 and possible health risks of offspring. J Reprod Immunol. 2021;143:1-8. DOI: 10.1016/j. jri.2020.103250

[41] Liu P, Zheng J, Yang P, Wang X, Wei C, Zhang S, et al. The immunologic status of newborns born to SARS-CoV-2-infected mothers in Wuhan, China. J Allergy Clin Immunol [Internet]. 2020;146(1):101-9. DOI: 10.1016/j. jaci.2020.04.038

[42] Zaigham M, Andersson O. Maternal and perinatal outcomes with COVID-19: A systematic review of 108 pregnancies. Acta Obstet Gynecol Scand. 2020;99(7):823-9. DOI: 10.1111/ aogs.13867

[43] Zimmermann P, Curtis N. COVID-19 in children, pregnancy and neonates: a review of epidemiologic and clinical features. Pediatr Infect Dis J.

2020;39(6):469-77. DOI: 10.1097/
INF.0000000000002700

[44] Berger JR. COVID-19 and the
nervous system. J Neurovirol.
2020;26:143-8. DOI: 10.1007/
s13365-020-00840-5

[45] Kim Y, Walser SA, Asghar SJ, Jain R,
Mainali G, Kumar A. A Comprehensive
review of neurologic manifestations of
COVID-19 and management of pre-
existing neurologic disorders in
children. J Child Neurol. 2021;36(4):
324-30. DOI: 10.1177/0883073820
968995

Toxic Stress Affecting Families and Children during the COVID-19 Pandemic: A Global Mental Health Crisis and an Emerging International Health Security Threat

Laura Czulada, Kevin M. Kover, Gabrielle Gracias, Kushee-Nidhi Kumar, Shanaya Desai, Stanislaw P. Stawicki, Kimberly Costello and Laurel Erickson-Parsons

Abstract

The coronavirus disease 2019 (COVID-19) pandemic has created numerous risk factors for families and children to experience toxic stress (TS). The widespread implementation of lockdowns and quarantines contributed to the increased incidence of domestic abuse and mental health issues while reducing opportunities for effective action, including social and educational interventions. Exposure to TS negatively affects a child's development which may result in a lasting impact on the child's life, as measured by tools, such as Adverse Childhood Experiences (ACE) score. When TS becomes highly prevalent within a society, it may develop into a health security threat, both from short- and long-term perspectives. Specific resources to combat the pandemic have been put in place, such as COVID-19 vaccines, novel therapeutics, and the use of telemedicine. However, the overall implementation has been challenging due to a multitude of factors, and more effort must be devoted to addressing issues that directly or indirectly lead to the emergence of TS. Only then can we begin to reduce the incidence and intensity of pandemic-associated toxic stress.

Keywords: coronavirus disease 2019, COVID-19, pandemic, Pediatrics, toxic stress

1. Introduction

Since its emergence more than 2 years ago, the coronavirus disease 2019 (COVID-19) pandemic has resulted in unprecedented stress for families around the world [1], and perhaps even more so for children [2]. Designed to help curtail the spread of the causative coronavirus, various "curve-flattening" measures have disrupted and/or distorted traditional social networks [3]. In this context, the stress in the absence of protective relationships can quickly become toxic, harming one's mental and physical health [4]. Interpersonal connections enable the conveyance of compassion and empathy. Without the presence of the above, individual development and well-being are likely to be negatively affected. This chapter discusses the topic of toxic stress (TS) among families and children during the current pandemic, focusing on identifying risk factors and deriving pragmatic solutions. These considerations are further superimposed on the relevance of TS to the general area of international health security, both in the short- and long-term timescales.

2. The coronavirus disease 2019 (COVID-19) pandemic

In Wuhan, Hubei Province, China in December 2019, pneumonia of an unknown origin started affecting index cases linked to a local wholesale food market [5]. Respiratory samples collected from these patients were subjected to genomic analysis, and the virus responsible was discovered to be a novel coronavirus related to Severe Acute Respiratory Syndrome Coronavirus (SARS-CoV). It was therefore named SARS-CoV-2, and the disease it causes was named coronavirus disease 2019 (COVID-19) [3, 5]. Due to its high infectivity, the novel coronavirus began spreading rapidly around the globe, leading the World Health Organization (WHO) to declare COVID-19 as a pandemic disease in March 2020 [6]. As of July 3, 2021, the total number of cases of COVID-19 in the United States was 33,530,880, including 15,555 new cases [7]. To date, more than 1,000,000 patients have died from COVID-19 in the United States alone [7].

In comparison, the 1918 Spanish influenza pandemic was caused by the H1N1 influenza A virus and lasted from 1918 to 1920 [8]. It disproportionately affected healthy, 25-40 years old individuals, who accounted for 40% of mortalities. By the end, the H1N1 pandemic was responsible for 50 million deaths worldwide [8]. In contrast, COVID-19 primarily affects people over the age of 65, especially those with comorbidities [8]. Although the overall mortality rate is very similar between the two pandemics - 2.5% for H1N1 and 2.4% for SARS-CoV2 - the mechanisms for mortality differ [8]. Whereas H1N1 tended to cause secondary bacterial pneumonia, SARS-CoV-2 resulted in an overactive immune response resulting in multiple organ failures [8]. The mean time to death for the H1N1 influenza was 2 weeks whereas it is 25 days for SARS-CoV2 [9, 10]. The latter finding is also responsible for the significant resource utilization (including intensive care utilization) related to COVID-19 cases.

Similar to the 1918 H1N1 pandemic, governments across the world implemented lockdown and quarantine strategies to contain the spread of COVID-19 [11]. In early 2020, many countries started implementing stay-at-home orders and sometimes more extensive shutdowns that mandated the closure of all non-essential businesses with concurrent stay-at-home orders to help minimize the spread of COVID-19 and to prevent hospitals from being overrun with COVID-19 patients [6, 12]. Additionally, universal masking mandates were put in place and there were physical distancing rules to maintain interpersonal distance of at least 6 feet between individuals when in public [5]. While these measures helped to contain the spread of COVID-19, they also had negative public health effects related to adverse childhood experiences (ACE, see later section) as well as TS [6].

3. Toxic stress risk factors and downstream sequelae: assessing the impact on health security

The SARS-CoV-2 pandemic has sent unprecedented shockwaves of stress through the global society. Severe stress in the absence of protective relationships may quickly escalate to become toxic, impairing both physical and mental health [13, 14].

Toxic stress is especially harmful to children, whose developing bodies and brains are highly susceptible to its negative effects, with potential long-term consequences [4]. Curve-flattening measures, including widespread school closures and social distancing, have disrupted the relational networks of billions of children around the globe [15]. Such disruptions, in conjunction with the severe economic stress caused by the pandemic, represent a once-in-a-century social crisis in the making [3]. Health security impacts will likely be felt for years if not decades to come, and will likely involve multiple domains that were previously defined in the ACAIM International Health Security Consensus [16].

Pandemics, armed conflict, and various forms of displacement pose a threat to the health and well-being of vulnerable populations and especially children [17]. As the global community begins to recognize the cumulative effects of various social and economic stressors related to the pandemic, the attention of researchers has shifted to TS and its short- and long-term health effects. Toxic stress, regarded as the result of prolonged activation of the stress response, can occur before birth and during childhood and is known to contribute to epigenetic changes, with potential health and neurodevelopmental consequences [18, 19]. Domestic abuse and child witnessed violence, both of which have increased during the pandemic, can further exacerbate the problem [3, 20–22]. However, various social factors and early and appropriate intervention can help mitigate many of the negative effects. We will now shift our focus to ACEs and their downstream consequences.

4. Adverse childhood experiences: focus on long-term sequelae

There exists a broad, fairly heterogeneous, and increasingly more recognized group of negative modulators of child well-being. Collectively, these events can be grouped under the umbrella of ACEs [23]. ACEs can stem from traumatic occurrences, and not infrequently may result in adverse downstream effects, both in physical and psychological/mental health domains. These traumatic experiences, among many, include poverty, physical/mental abuse, mental illness, and community violence [23–25]. When multiple ACEs occur together there is a much greater probability of the child experiencing long-term health effects [26]. To investigate the relationship between ACEs and negative health outcomes, a study was conducted, surveying adults in San Diego, California, about their childhood history to determine if there was a correlation between ACEs and future health conditions [27, 28]. The study indicated that early emotional trauma may indeed be associated with future adverse health consequences [27]. This, in turn, suggests that traumatic experiences in childhood may pose a long-term threat to our health systems and therefore broadly understood health security. More specifically, ACEs, especially if repeated/recurring, may be associated with a higher prevalence of cancer, depression, and other chronic diseases [26, 29–31]. However, a child experiencing ACEs may not necessarily equate to future long-term adverse health effects [26]. This in part, is due to the resiliency of the child, their ability to cope with traumatic experiences, and their overall support structure [26]. In the context of the COVID-19 pandemic, the latter may also be significantly affected, resulting in loss of critical social support for the child experiencing ACEs.

Another 2021 study published in BMC Public Health showed a correlation between ACEs and self-rated health (SRH) in young adults [32]. In this prospective cohort study of ACE exposure, ACEs were tracked at varying age groups and SRH values were also recorded for comparison. There was a proportional increase in ACE and SRH scores [32], suggesting a substantial degree of correlation. A better understanding of ACEs may lead to more accurate approaches for predicting future health effects of ACEs and, therefore, may help in the development of earlier and more effective interventions. As such, this general strategy may be one of the key components of addressing health security concerns related to downstream sequelae of ACEs.

Based on existing evidence, early intervention is critical when approaching ACEs to minimize their long-term, negative effects. The Centers for Disease Control and Prevention (CDC) suggest six strategies to reduce ACEs: strengthening economic support for families; promoting social norms that protect against violence and adversity; ensuring strong starts for children; enhancing skills to help parents and youth handle stress; managing emotions; as well as tackling everyday challenges, connecting youth to caring adults and activities, and intervening to lessen immediate and long-term harms [33]. However, with the COVID-19 pandemic, there has been an increase in occurrences of ACEs due to the lockdowns and quarantines implemented to help stop the spread of SARS-CoV-2 [34]. The lockdowns are forcing some children to stay in homes that are emotionally unhealthy and traumatic [34]. Additionally, the lockdowns have also made it more difficult to implement many of the strategies that the CDC suggests are needed to prevent ACEs [15].

5. Mental health trends in the pandemic: exploring long term impacts on health security

The COVID-19 pandemic has had many negative effects on the mental health of both adults and children [35, 36]. The stress associated with the fear of the unknown, along with the abrupt closure of schools in March 2020, spiraled many children into emotional upheavals they had not experienced previously. The sudden switch from "going to work" every day to "working from home" or being furloughed or laid off led to enormous financial stress for many families. Not feeling financially secure may lead to significant emotional pressure for adults, which is often projected onto children, in various and often unpredictable ways. The closure of schools and businesses resulted in a significant reduction in direct human contact. Casual daily social interactions constitute an important outlet for mental health stress for many people [37, 38].

Prior to the pandemic, approximately 1 in 10 adults reported anxiety or depressive disorder. This increased during the pandemic, with about 4 in 10 adults reporting corresponding symptoms [10]. A survey in June 2020 showed that 13% of adults admitted to increased or new substance use, attributing such response to the stress related to the COVID-19 pandemic [10]. It is well established that mental health stress in adults directly impacts toxic stress in children [39, 40]. When adults are under stress, they have less emotional "reserve" or "bandwidth" to effectively care for their children, which may, in turn, result in physical child abuse, emotional child abuse, neglect, or unhealthy interactions that although not necessarily outright abusive, may still have deleterious effects on our children [41, 42].

Irritability, inattention, and clinginess were seen among children in early pandemic studies along with sleep issues, decreased appetite, and separation anxiety [43]. Adolescents may be prone to hoarding behavior due to the panic-buying seen in the early pandemic. Obsessive–compulsive behavior may be increased because of hoarding, general feelings of fear and uncertainty, a heightened awareness of how viruses are spread, as well as the need for cleanliness to prevent viral spread [43]. Increased reliance on electronic devices for online schooling or as a means for human interaction while in the quarantine may lead to worsening social media/electronic addiction as well as cyberbullying [43, 44].

The mental health needs of our society related to the COVID-19 pandemic, will continue to be apparent for years to come. Many downstream effects will be unpredictable, individualized, and likely highly variable in terms of temporal patterns. Toxic stress from the poor mental health of our adults and children will lead to deleterious emotional and health effects that are yet to be seen. Focusing on the mental health of our entire population is essential to help decrease these effects. Increased mental health support with both inpatient and outpatient resources is needed now, and will certainly be needed for the foreseeable future.

6. Toxic stress as an international health security threat

No one is immune to the effects of COVID-19. In addition to millions of confirmed cases worldwide, COVID-19's effects on individuals and communities extend far beyond hospitalizations, morbidity, and mortality. Pandemics have deleterious consequences on the well-being of individuals and communities through direct effects of the illness and emotional isolation, economic loss, work and school closures, and maldistribution of resources [45]. Published data describe how various consequences of pandemic mitigation efforts (such as quarantine) affect stress, depression, fear, anger, boredom, stigma, and other negative states. Adults readily report worse psychological well-being now as compared to before the pandemic [46]. Because data suggest that children might less frequently transmit or become severely ill from the virus, the more unique consequences that COVID-19 has on children may easily be overlooked. Although data on child and family well-being during COVID-19 are not as robust, increasing reports of intimate partner and family violence around the globe continue to be of great concern [47–49]. Long-term impacts on broadly defined health security will likely be both significant and difficult to predict.

Within the international context, conflict-affected populations are particularly vulnerable to COVID-19. Overcrowding and inadequate water and sanitation systems in refugee camps and informal settlements, coupled with previously existing illnesses, may increase the spread of COVID-19 and further exacerbate the emotional trauma upon the most vulnerable segments of the population. Moreover, resource and health system constraints may restrict access to adequate and appropriate care. Control measures such as physical distancing may be difficult and may also increase economic precarity, intimate partner violence, and food insecurity in populations already vulnerable [3]. The incidence of post-traumatic stress will likely increase following the pandemic – another "invisible" aspect of this global event, reported following previous emerging infectious disease outbreaks [50].

Downstream, long-term consequences of toxic stress are more poorly understood, but the associated increase in behavioral health issues, combined with secondary implications inherent to these considerations, are bound to create a truly global urgency and crisis [4, 51]. This is especially true when looking at geographic areas with limited resources and a lack of robust mental health infrastructure. In terms of addressing some of the challenges related to halting any downstream escalations secondary to toxic stress, several truly international strategies can be considered. Among those, the most prominent is telehealth/telemedicine, as discussed in a subsequent section of this chapter [52, 53]. Other important components here include the provision of safe environments, education, as well as ongoing close support and reassurance.

7. Vaccination availability: a gateway to normalcy

On December 14, 2020, the U.S. COVID-19 Vaccination Program began, with vaccines from Pfizer (New York, NY); Moderna (Cambridge, MA); and Johnson & Johnson (New Brunswick, NJ) being deployed [54], first for domestic then for global use. To date, Pfizer and Moderna each require two shots to achieve fully immunized status, whereas Johnson & Johnson requires a single shot [55]. Pfizer vaccines must be given to patients ages 12 and older, while Moderna and Johnson & Johnson vaccines must be given to patients ages 18 and up [55]. An additional booster dose has been recommended by all companies for patients ages 12 and up [55]. Other countries also deployed their own vaccines to meet local needs [56]. As of April 1, 2022, as many as 561,173,692 COVID-19 vaccines have been administered (255,582,575 have received at least one dose and 217,703,007 are fully vaccinated); thus, 77% of the U.S. population has received one dose, and 65.6% are fully vaccinated [54]. Studies have shown that Pfizer and Moderna vaccines are approximately 94-95% effective for patients who have received the second dose and 64% for those who have received just one dose [57]. The Johnson & Johnson vaccine has shown 66.3% effectiveness in clinical trials for patients with no prior COVID-19 infection [58]. Compared to fully vaccinated patients, unvaccinated children are 1.6 to 2 times more likely to be hospitalized, and adults are 5 times more likely to be hospitalized [55]. According to the CDC, the number of new COVID-19 hospital admissions has been generally decreasing from April 19 to June 22, 2021 [55]. Therefore, the global distribution of COVID-19 vaccinations appears to be providing immunity against the virus, shown by the decline in hospitalization and a slower increase in new cases of COVID-19.

Increased vaccination rates in eligible candidates significantly help to curb virus transmission rates within a population. This, in turn, may be able help neighborhoods to lift quarantine and lockdown measures, aid in a quicker return to "normal", which therefore may help reduce the toxic stressful environment and its harmful consequences on children. Consequently, well-implemented vaccination programs are critical to international health security, the well-being of the global population inclusive of children, as well as our current best attempt at the return to normalcy [59].

8. Role of telemedicine: an important part of a comprehensive mitigation framework

Telemedicine plays an important role in our collective efforts to prevent and mitigate toxic childhood stress in the COVID-19 era [52, 60]. By leveraging technology to deliver patient care remotely, telemedicine enables interpersonal connectivity while overcoming many of the limitations related to either social distancing or lack of resources (e.g., transportation). Health care providers, through virtual visits and other telehealth platforms, may be able to provide effective emotional support and psychosocial buffering for families experiencing acute stress [61].

Through the provision of frequent interpersonal touchpoints, telemedicine can furnish an important platform to support the well-being of children [62]. One of telemedicine's main strengths resides in the ability to reduce costs associated with access to care, primarily by reducing the time and expense of travel, waiting, and paid time off [63, 64]. Moreover, health systems can leverage the lower associated cost(s) to perform more frequent virtual check-ins (and thus provide more support). More face-to-face time, in turn, helps build trust and creates opportunities for providers to affirm families' strengths and resiliencies, as well as reinforce strategies that are effective in combating acute stress, including balanced nutrition, physical activity, quality sleep, mindfulness practices, supportive relationships, and mental health care [65–67].

In the wake of widespread parental fears regarding the potential for exposure of children to COVID-19, telemedicine can help make all stakeholders feel safer, especially in terms of public immunization programs. This is a very important aspect of the overall care provision since visit volume in many outpatient pediatric offices decreased by >50% and vaccine orders have fallen by 2.5 million since March 2020 [68]. The American Academy of Pediatrics has urged the continued provision of routine immunizations for children. In response, some practices have begun offering curbside and drive-through immunization clinics [68]. Utilizing telemedicine for interpersonal connection and relationship building alongside socially distanced medical procedures such as immunizations and biometrics could help optimize the balance between putting patients at ease and bringing them up to date with care.

Telemedicine has its limitations in evaluating the well-being of children and parents. Establishing and maintaining a personal connection with a family is more easily done with an in-person visit. Signs of child abuse may be missed as physical exams are limited during a telemedicine visit. Bruising and intentional skin trauma may not be appreciated through a camera. Intraoral trauma would be difficult to identify [69]. It is more difficult to speak with children alone through a virtual visit and they may be less willing to identify stressors with parents present [69]. Mental health evaluation may be challenging if children do not feel comfortable divulging information while at home or in front of their parents. In contrast with in-person visits, where those present are seen and accounted for, situational awareness during virtual visits is more limited. For example, a violent partner or parent could be present during a virtual visit but out of audio or video range. Traditional social screening questions such as "do you feel safe at home?" may not only have lower utility in a virtual visit, but they could also risk exacerbating household tensions [61].

In light of the above considerations, approaches aimed at specific educational initiatives have been proposed by domestic violence and toxic stress experts during the COVID-19 pandemic. Beyond virtual visits, advances in telemedicine could empower patients through easily (and confidentially) accessible information and resources [61]. Other helpful tools could include confidential two-way messaging platforms and clinical message pools for providers to streamline referrals. Provider education models, such as Safe Environment for Every Kid (i.e., seekwellbeing. org), which incorporate social work collaboration, have been shown to effectively prevent child maltreatment. Trauma-informed screening tools, such as the Pediatric Adverse Childhood Experiences and Related Life-event Screener, have demonstrated strong face validity in pediatric primary care [28]. Adopting such approaches to the telemedicine space could be highly promising. Various sets of specific considerations applicable to health security may also be applicable 'by proxy' due to the benefits gained via telemedicine-based behavioral health interventions.

9. Conclusion

The COVID-19 pandemic has ushered dramatic social and economic upheavals, leading to a highly stressful period in our history, especially challenging for families and children. The identification and prevention of toxic childhood stress in the COVID-19 era may be especially difficult during this time. Much remains to be learned about risk factors and ways to remediate this serious health security threat, especially when considering its potential long-term consequences. The initial steps to begin healing our children from a hopefully once-in-a-lifetime pandemic include: 1) widespread recognition and identification of the effects of toxic stress on children, as measured by validated tools, such as Adverse Childhood Event (ACE) scores, and its possible impact on the development of chronic diseases and mental health issues later in life; 2) increase in vaccination rates across all eligible candidate groups; and 3) implementation of telemedicine to support access to health needs, and to build and maintain relationships between healthcare workers and the community. Although the implementation of the above steps may be challenging, continued support and necessary resources must be put forth toward one of our most vulnerable populations to help remediate the long-lasting impact of TS for years to come.

Author details

Laura Czulada[1], Kevin M. Kover[2], Gabrielle Gracias[3], Kushee-Nidhi Kumar[4], Shanaya Desai[4], Stanislaw P. Stawicki[4*], Kimberly Costello[1] and Laurel Erickson-Parsons[1]

1 Department of Pediatrics, St. Luke's University Health Network, Bethlehem, Pennsylvania, USA

2 Philadelphia College of Osteopathic Medicine, Philadelphia, Pennsylvania, USA

3 Lehigh University, Bethlehem, Pennsylvania, USA

4 Department of Research and Innovation, St. Luke's University Health Network, Bethlehem, Pennsylvania, USA

*Address all correspondence to: stawicki.ace@gmail.com

IntechOpen

References

[1] Rudolph CW, Zacher H. Family demands and satisfaction with family life during the COVID-19 pandemic. Couple and Family Psychology: Research and Practice. 2021:**10**(4): 249-259

[2] Halty L, Halty A, de Gregorio VC. Support for families during COVID-19 in Spain: The iCygnus online tool for parents. Child Psychiatry & Human Development. 2021;**4**:1-14

[3] Stawicki SP et al. The 2019-2020 novel coronavirus (severe acute respiratory syndrome coronavirus 2) pandemic: A joint american college of academic international medicine-world academic council of emergency medicine multidisciplinary COVID-19 working group consensus paper. Journal of Global Infectious Diseases. 2020;**12**(2):47

[4] Shonkoff JP et al. The lifelong effects of early childhood adversity and toxic stress. Pediatrics. 2012;**129**(1):e232-e246

[5] Ciotti M et al. The COVID-19 pandemic. Critical Reviews in Clinical Laboratory Sciences. 2020;**57**(6): 365-388

[6] Singh J, Singh J. COVID-19 and Its Impact on Society Electronic Research Journal of Social Sciences and Humanities. 2020:**2**(1):168-172

[7] CDC. CDC COVID Data Tracker. 2021. Available from: https://covid.cdc.gov/covid-data-tracker/#cases_casesper100k. [Accessed: July 14, 2021]

[8] Liang ST, Liang LT, Rosen JM. COVID-19: A comparison to the 1918 influenza and how we can defeat it. Postgraduate Medical Journal. 2021;**97**(1147):273-274

[9] Mills CE, Robins JM, Lipsitch M. Transmissibility of 1918 pandemic influenza. Nature. 2004;**432**(7019): 904-906

[10] Panchal N, Kamal R, Cox C, Garfield R. The Implications of COVID-19 for Mental Health and Substance Use. Vol. 21. Kaiser Family Foundation (KFF); 2020

[11] Benke C et al. Lockdown, quarantine measures, and social distancing: Associations with depression, anxiety and distress at the beginning of the COVID-19 pandemic among adults from Germany. Psychiatry Research. 2020;**293**:113462

[12] Ratnasekera AM, Seng SS, Jacovides CL, et al. Rising incidence of interpersonal violence in Pennsylvania during COVID-19 stay-at home order. Surgery. 2022;**171**(2):533-540

[13] Johnson SB et al. The science of early life toxic stress for pediatric practice and advocacy. Pediatrics. 2013;**131**(2):319-327

[14] Garner AS. Home visiting and the biology of toxic stress: Opportunities to address early childhood adversity. Pediatrics. 2013;**132**(Suppl. 2):S65-S73

[15] Papadimos TJ et al. COVID-19 blind spots: A consensus statement on the importance of competent political leadership and the need for public health cognizance. Journal of Global Infectious Diseases. 2020;**12**(4):167

[16] Le NK et al. International health security: A summative assessment by ACAIM consensus group. In: Contemporary Developments and Perspectives in International Health Security. Vol. 1. London, UK: IntechOpen; 2020

[17] Le NK et al. What's new in academic international medicine? International health security agenda–expanded and

re-defined. International Journal of Academic Medicine. 2020;**6**(3):163

[18] Bergman NJ. Birth practices: Maternal-neonate separation as a source of toxic stress. Birth Defects Research. 2019;**111**(15):1087-1109

[19] Ridout KK, Khan M, Ridout SJ. Adverse childhood experiences run deep: Toxic early life stress, telomeres, and mitochondrial DNA copy number, the biological markers of cumulative stress. BioEssays. 2018;**40**(9):1800077

[20] Tsavoussis A et al. Child-witnessed domestic violence and its adverse effects on brain development: A call for societal self-examination and awareness. Frontiers in Public Health. 2014;**2**:178

[21] Tsavoussis A, Stawicki SP, Papadimos TJ. Child-witnessed domestic violence: An epidemic in the shadows. International Journal of Critical Illness and Injury Science. 2015;**5**(1):64

[22] Hon HH et al. What's new in critical illness and injury science? Nonaccidental burn injuries, child abuse awareness and prevention, and the critical need for dedicated pediatric emergency specialists: Answering the global call for social justice for our youngest citizens. International Journal of Critical Illness and Injury Science. 2015;**5**(4):223

[23] Benson KL. Teacher Training for Students Affected by Adverse Childhood Experiences (ACEs). California Lutheran University ProQuest Dissertations Publishing; 2020

[24] Bartlett JD, Sacks V. Adverse Childhood Experiences Are Different than Child Trauma, and it's Critical to Understand Why. Available online at: https://www.rdn.bc.ca/sites/default/files/2020-10/adverse_childhood_experiences.pdf Last accessed on May 20, 2022

[25] Greeson JK et al. Traumatic childhood experiences in the 21st century: Broadening and building on the ACE studies with data from the National Child Traumatic Stress Network. Journal of Interpersonal Violence. 2014;**29**(3):536-556

[26] Crouch E et al. Safe, stable, and nurtured: Protective factors against poor physical and mental health outcomes following exposure to adverse childhood experiences (ACEs). Journal of Child & Adolescent Trauma. 2019;**12**(2): 165-173

[27] Felitti VJ. The relation between adverse childhood experiences and adult health: Turning gold into lead. The Permanente Journal. 2002;**6**(1):44

[28] Boullier M, Blair M. Adverse childhood experiences. Paediatrics and Child Health. 2018;**28**(3):132-137

[29] Dube SR et al. Cumulative childhood stress and autoimmune diseases in adults. Psychosomatic Medicine. 2009;**71**(2):243

[30] Middlebrooks JS, Audage NC. The Effects of Childhood Stress on Health across the Lifespan. National Center for Injury Prevention and Control of the Centers for Disease. CDC Stacks Public Health Publications; 2008

[31] Alvarez J et al. The relationship between child abuse and adult obesity among California women. American Journal of Preventive Medicine. 2007;**33**(1):28-33

[32] Jahn A et al. Adverse childhood experiences and future self-rated health: A prospective cohort study. BMC Public Health. 2021;**21**(1):1-11

[33] Jones C, Bacon S, Myers G, Kacha-Ochana A, Mahmood A. National Center for Injury Prevention and Control Adverse Childhood Experiences Prevention Strategy FY2021-FY2024.

CDC Stacks Public Health Publications. 2020

[34] Bryant DJ, Oo M, Damian AJ. The rise of adverse childhood experiences during the COVID-19 pandemic. Psychological Trauma. 2020;**12**(S1): S193-S194

[35] Kwong AS et al. Mental health before and during the COVID-19 pandemic in two longitudinal UK population cohorts. The British Journal of Psychiatry. 2021;**218**(6):334-343

[36] Hoekstra PJ. Suicidality in children and adolescents: Lessons to be learned from the COVID-19 crisis. Eur Child Adolesc Psychiatry. 2020;**29**(6):737-738

[37] Das S. Mental health and psychosocial aspects of COVID-19 in India: The challenges and responses. Journal of Health Management. 2020;**22**(2):197-205

[38] Singh S, Roy D, Sinha K, Parveen S, Sharma G, Joshi G. Impact of COVID-19 and lockdown on mental health of children and adolescents: A narrative review with recommendations. Psychiatry research. 2020;**293**:113429

[39] McEwen CA, McEwen BS. Social structure, adversity, toxic stress, and intergenerational poverty: An early childhood model. Annual Review of Sociology. 2017;**43**:445-472

[40] Shern DL, Blanch AK, Steverman SM. Toxic stress, behavioral health, and the next major era in public health. American Journal of Orthopsychiatry. 2016;**86**(2):109

[41] Jakob P. Multi-stressed families, child violence and the larger system: An adaptation of the nonviolent model. Journal of Family Therapy. 2018;**40**(1): 25-44

[42] Silvern L. Parenting and family stress as mediators of the long-term

effects of child abuse. Child Abuse & Neglect. 1994;**18**(5):439-453

[43] Singh S, Roy D, Sinha K, Parveen S, Sharma G, Joshi G. Impact of COVID-19 and lockdown on mental health of children and adolescents: A narrative review with recommendations. Psychiatry research. 2020;**293**:113429

[44] Stawicki SP, Firstenberg MS, Papadimos TJ. The growing role of social media in international health security: The good, the bad, and the ugly. In: Global Health Security. Springer; 2020:341-357

[45] Janssen LH et al. Does the COVID-19 pandemic impact parents' and adolescents' well-being? An EMA-study on daily affect and parenting. PLoS One. 2020;**15**(10):e0240962

[46] Morrow-Howell N, Galucia N, Swinford E. Recovering from the COVID-19 pandemic: A focus on older adults. Journal of Aging & Social Policy. 2020;**32**(4-5):526-535

[47] Humphreys KL. Myint MT, Zeanah CH. Increased Risk for Family Violence During the COVID-19 Pandemic. Pediatrics. 2020;**146**(1):e20200982

[48] Zhang H. The influence of the ongoing COVID-19 pandemic on family violence in China. Journal of Family Violence. 2020;**9**:1-11

[49] Usher K, Bhullar N, Durkin J, Gyamfi N, Jackson D. Family violence and COVID-19: Increased vulnerability and reduced options for support. International Journal of Mental Health Nursing. 2020;**29**(4):549-552

[50] Paladino L et al. Reflections on the Ebola public health emergency of international concern, part 2: The unseen epidemic of posttraumatic stress among health-care personnel and survivors of the 2014-2016 Ebola outbreak. Journal of Global Infectious Diseases. 2017;**9**(2):45

[51] Franke HA. Toxic stress: Effects, prevention and treatment. Children. 2014;**1**(3):390-402

[52] Chauhan V et al. Novel coronavirus (COVID-19): Leveraging telemedicine to optimize care while minimizing exposures and viral transmission. Journal of Emergencies, Trauma, and Shock. 2020;**13**(1):20

[53] Kelley KC et al. Answering the challenge of COVID-19 pandemic through innovation and ingenuity. Advances in Experimental Medicine and Biology. 2021;**1318**:859-873

[54] CDC. COVID Data Tracker Weekly Review. 2021. Available from: www.cdc. gov/coronavirus/2019-ncov/covid-data/ covidview/index.html [Accessed: July 14, 2021]

[55] CDC. Different COVID-19 Vaccines. 2021. Available from: https://www.cdc. gov/coronavirus/2019-ncov/vaccines/ different-vaccines.html [Accessed: July 14, 2021]

[56] Baraniuk C. How to vaccinate the world against covid-19. BMJ (Clinical research ed.). 2021;**372**, n211

[57] Pfizer-BioNTech and Moderna vaccines against COVID-19 among hospitalized adults aged ≥ 65 years— United States, January–march 2021. MMWR. Morbidity and Mortality Weekly Report; 2021;**70**(18):674-679

[58] CDC, Johnson & Johnson's Janssen COVID-19 Vaccine Overview and Safety (2021). 2021, April

[59] Shayak B, Sharma MM. COVID-19 spreading dynamics with vaccination-allocation strategy. Return to Normalcy and Vaccine Hesitancy. medRxiv. 2020;**1**:1-23.

[60] Chauhan V et al. State of the globe: The trials and tribulations of the COVID-19 pandemic: Separated but together, telemedicine revolution, frontline struggle against "silent hypoxia," the relentless search for novel therapeutics and vaccines, and the daunting prospect of "COVIFLU". Journal of Global Infectious Diseases. 2020;**12**(2):39

[61] Bottino CJ. Preventing toxic childhood stress in the COVID era: A role for telemedicine. Telemedicine and e-Health. 2021;**27**(4):385-387

[62] Goldschmidt K. The COVID-19 Pandemic: Technology use to Support the Wellbeing of Children. Journal of Pediatric Nursing. 2020;**53**:88-90

[63] Speedie SM et al. Telehealth: The promise of new care delivery models. Telemedicine and e-Health. 2008;**14**(9):964-967

[64] Institute of Medicine (US) Committee on Evaluating Clinical Applications of Telemedicine. In: Field MJ, editor. Telemedicine: A Guide to Assessing Telecommunications in Health Care. Washington (DC): National Academies Press (US); 1996

[65] Aware A. ACEs AWARE MASTER FAQ

[66] Briguglio M et al. Healthy eating, physical activity, and sleep hygiene (HEPAS) as the winning triad for sustaining physical and mental health in patients at risk for or with neuropsychiatric disorders: Considerations for clinical practice. Neuropsychiatric Disease and Treatment. 2020;**16**:55

[67] Prakash J et al. Role of various lifestyle and behavioral strategies in positive mental health across a preventive to therapeutic continuum. Industrial Psychiatry Journal. 2020;**29**(2):185

[68] Bramer CA et al. Decline in child vaccination coverage during the COVID-19 pandemic—Michigan care

improvement registry, May 2016-May
2020. American Journal of
Transplantation. 2020;**20**(7):1930

[69] Racine N et al. Telemental health for
child trauma treatment during and
post-COVID-19: Limitations and
considerations. Child Abuse & Neglect.
2020;**110**:104698

A Journey through and beyond the COVID-19 Pandemic in Indian Setup-Lessons Learnt So Far

Divyesh Kumar

Abstract

World over life was going at its normal pace when an outbreak occurred in Hubei province of China in the later part of the year 2019. This outbreak was soon found to be caused by a virus named coronavirus (COVID-19). Rapidly the virus spread globally leading to a pandemic. The mortality rate was increasing day by day and helplessly everyone was wondering what actually could be done to prevent the spread. Lessons from the past epidemic made it possible to think that maintaining social distancing and adequate hygiene might help to combat the ailment. In India, majorly affected were the people from poor strata and the businessmen who were earning their daily bread by selling things of daily need. The health sector too witnessed an alarming ratio of patients suffering from COVID-19. The second wave, which soon followd the first wave, caused much more havoc. Overall, the COVID-19 pandemic, exposed and challanged the health security system of every country. As the danger of pandemic still prevails, steps to curtail the spread of disease and future management strategies should be formulated from the lessons learnt through the COVID-19 phase.

Keywords: COVID-19, Lessons, India

1. Introduction

The year 2019 started with a bang and happiness, with colourful crackers exploding in the sky. Everything throughout the year went at its normal rhythm with the later part of the year bringing some bad news from the Hubei region in China. There was news of a spread of a deadly virus, which was found to be caused by the coronavirus. It was sooner found to affect people from other parts of the world, suggesting human-to-human transmission [1]. WHO declared it a public health emergency on March 11, 2020 [2].

The coronavirus disease (COVID-19) was found to affect the respiratory tract and also was found to affect the gastrointestinal tract and other parts of the body. Although symptoms vary from person to person, the major symptoms were found to be cough, fever, headache, sore throat, and diarrhoea [3]. Besides symptomatic patients majority of the spread was due to the asymptomatic carriers, which without any symptoms harboured the disease and were the major culprit in the spread of the disease.

Ever since there has been an outbreak of the COVID-19 from China, besides a lot many casualties, the economic front has also been shattered due to lockdown, worldwide. The COVID-19 disease not only affected the healthcare sector but also has had a deep impact on the tourism and trade sector worldwide [4], which has made the economy take a backseat.

Hence, urgent steps need to be taken to bring back life to new normal; also, the lessons learned from the COVID-19 pandemic propels us to formulate guidelines to tackle future untoward events.

2. Journey through the COVID-19 pandemic phases in India and its impact on various sectors

2.1 The initial impact

Although the initial impact of the virus was seen majorly in the developed countries, India got affected during January when the first case of it was reported from the Kerala province in southern India [5].

Further, lockdown and curfew were imposed in different countries, which eventually dwindled the economy globally affecting the poor and middle-class earners, maximally. In India, the daily wagers were forced to flee from their working place to go back to their native places. Since transportation was at standstill due to lockdown these workers along with their family members had to cover their long distances on foot only. Sooner or later, many social activists took the initiative to help these sufferers. At this point, the blame game of the politicians towards each other started pouring in.

Over time, the COVID-19 pandemic has affected many sectors which majorly include health, education, hospitality, and entertainment sectors. Diagramatic representation as documented in **Figure 1**.

2.2 Impact on the health sector

The situation on the other hand, in the hospital sector, was far more frightening as more and more casualties were happening due to limited beds and a greater number of patients requiring hospitalisation. Urgent steps were thought of and many

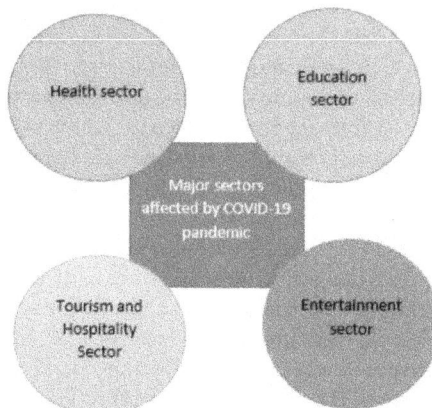

Figure 1.
Various sectors affected by the COVID-19 pandemic.

places like hotels, train bogies, etc. were soon made as alternatives to hospital beds. Health care workers despite all the stress of contracting the disease themselves took the front seat to take care of the sufferers, but to their very surprise many people, by this time, had become prey to different myths and false beliefs and had to face the resistance from these society members. The situation was grave in certain parts of the country and police had to take some harsh steps to control the nuisance.

Amongst the patients, the effect was seen majorly in elderlies and in patients suffering from cancer and with comorbidities. In their article published by Wang et al., concluded that patients above 70 years of age had a faster progression of disease in the elderlies [6]. Similarly, a study was done by Liang et al. documented that case-fatality rates were higher in elderlies and also the pulmonary complication requiring resuscitation were higher in those suffering from cancer [7]. Besides its impact on these patients treatment delays due to the lockdown became a major issue. Various modifications in the treatment guidelines were framed by this time by various eminent treating societies to make the treatment continued and minimise the delays. Also, working protocols of different departments were modified and policies to screen the COVID-19 patients were formulated.

Though modified protocols were important from the clinical point of view, the psychological effect of the suffering had a deep impact on society. Effective health-related communication has thus remained a need of the hour. An article published by A. Finset et al. concluded that effective health communication is important in fighting the COVID-19 pandemic [8]. Similar importance of health communication has been documented by Reddy et al. in their article [9]. Amongst the various modes of communication, telecommunication with patients has also proved to a boom during the pandemic. As the majority of the patients who had queries related to the disease and treatment-related queries were also taken care of. Also, scheduling of all appointments further made things organised both for the patients as well as the treating physicians.

From a treatment point of view the rat race to treat and cure the ailment was soon catching the pace by this time. Many different permutation and combinations of drugs were thought of during this phase, with not much success to it. Alternative medicines like homoeopathy and ayurvedic soon joined the race and tried their best to come up with a possible solution. Since the disease was due to the virus, the only hope for it was thought of by generating an appropriate vaccine. Research on making the vaccine soon began. Different countries to the very best of their capabilities are trying till date, to make an effective vaccine. In India, Bharat Biotech took the initiative and completed the initial phases of the trials.

Covaxin and Covishield are the two vaccines that were developed and brought forward for mass vaccination. The Government decided to carry out the vaccination in a phased manner with age group 45 and above along with health care workers and patients with comorbidities receiving the initial jab. Although a majority of people have got vaccinated, a lot many still doubt the efficacy of the vaccine and remain concerned with its side effects. The false rumours regarding the vaccine have further added to it and have prevented a lot of many to refrain from getting vaccinated. While people were being told about the advantages and necessity of getting the vaccination done, the second wave of the pandemic came into existence.

2.3 Impact of the COVID-19 on the education sector

The very initial phase of the COVID-19 pandemic deeply impacted the education front, as the lockdown and curfew forced all the schools, colleges, and universities to shut down. The digital model was soon implemented and the majority of the teaching soon began through online mode. An article published by Pravat Kumar Jena, has highlighted the various initiatives taken by the Govt. Of India on the education sector. Also various positive and negative effects have been emphasised [10].

Although the effect of this form of education can only be assessed with time as of now, the digital mode has surely taken care of the education front.

2.4 Impact of the COVID-19 on the tourism and hospitality sector

Besides the health and the education sector, the hospitality industry has also been affected badly by the pandemic. The hospitality industry accounts for 10% of the global GDP. The travel restrictions have not only led to revenue losses also the jobs of various workers have come to stake. As per United Nations World Tourism Organisation that international tourists will be down by 20–30%

In India, the hospitality industry is likely to be hit hard. Experts suggest that domestic hotel companies faced a weak FY20 and a much weaker FY21. The challenges and learnings from the COVID-19 pandemic in the Indian setting have been elaborated in the article published by V. Kaushal et al. [11].

Other than India, the major impact of the COVID-19 pandemic can also be seen in countries whose economy depends largely on the tourism and hospitality sector.

2.5 Impact of the COVID-19 on the entertainment sector

Music and film plays a very important role in one's life and is not only a source of entertainment but is also a major revenue generator for the country. The lockdown and curfew have led to the downfall in film production and indirectly to revenue collection. G. Nhamo et al. in their study found that the pandemic has led to the cancellation of productions, films, and music festivals leading to multibillionaire losses which furthermore has led to a devastating impact on the livelihood of artists [12].

2.6 COVID-19 and international health security

United Nations brought the concept of health security during the year 1994 [13]. Some of the alternative terms include global public health security, public health security, and global health security [14–18]. Global Health Security is defined as the activities required, both proactive and reactive, to minimise the danger and impact of acute public health events that endanger people's health across geographical regions and international boundaries [19]. Four well-known international organisations that takes care of the health security issues are- World Health Organisation (WHO), the United Nations (UN), the European Union (EU), and the Asia-Pacific Economic Cooperation (APEC).

A well-developed Health security system is the backbone of a strong infrastaructure of every country. The ongoing COVID-19 pandemic has shown how segregated and poorly funded health systems are worldwide. In a simplified form, it could be said that it has exposed the ground realities of the health security systems of all countries, revealing that no country is safe. Even countries like the USA, UK which receives top ratings for pandemic preparedness in the Global Health Security Index, have reported a significant number of COVID-19 cases and deaths [20]. India on the other hand, ranks at 57th position, with a cumulative score of 46.5, and fairs poor in the Global Health security index [21]. Compared to other countries, though the COVID-19 outbreak occurred late in India, the impact of it was much more severe. Further, the effect was seen in a wavy fashion with the first wave soon followed by the second wave. The impact of the second wave was much more severe than the first wave and majorly affected the younger population. Although India shares with the United Nations the Global Health Security Agenda (GHSA), still a lot many steps are needed to be taken to improvise the Health security status.

Furthermore, not always security concerns are overlapped with health issues. Recently, both bioterrorism and emerging infectious diseases have raised alarming bells on health security issues [22–24]. An international cooperation is thus highly solicited in containing the spread of infectious diseases and enforcing a strong health security system. Also, establishing a global centralised Disaster Management Society and developing a comprehensive Global Disaster Rescue Plan could be possible measures for curtailing future pandemics.

3. The second wave of COVID-19 pandemic

Although unlocking in phases was being attempted to resume the work situation as before, the casual attitude of people of not wearing a mask and maintaining proper hygiene once more has brought the second wave of the pandemic into the picture. The second wave although started gradually but sooner has spread at a great speed throughout the country, with the majority of the cases being reported from Maharashtra, Uttar Pradesh, and New Delhi.

A decline of the active cases was noticed until Feb-March 2021 when a sudden rise of cases began to be noticed. So, who actually can be blamed for this sudden sprout of the diseases for the second time? Crowded election rallies, religious and other social gatherings, and early opening of public places are being considered as the causative factors for the spread of the disease. India is a country of diversity and is highly populated with a variation of people ranging from very poor to very rich. The most affected group is the lower strata of people.

Hence complete lockdown probably was never an answer. The casual attitude of the countrymen towards the disease is the only factor that probably has led to this second wave. The situation has worsened this time as the rate of casualties has taken a steep rise, hospital facilities are full, and demand for oxygen and medications has increased from before.

A new double mutant variant of the coronavirus has been detected from the collected samples from different states of the country. B.1.617 lineage is known as the 'double mutant' virus. An increase in the fraction of samples with the E484Q and L452R mutations he been found by the Indian SARS-CoV-2 Consortium on Genomics (INSACOG) group. Besides.

India some other countries like the US, UK, Denmark, and Switzerland have also come across similar mutant strains. A new lineage of the SARS-CoV-2 virus, called B.1.618, has been identified in West Bengal, India.

Since the vaccine has remained the only hope of tackling the virus, scientists world over are trying their level best to develop an effective vaccine. Sputnik V vaccine is the latest one and has shown effective results in the trials done, so far. In their interim analysis report, Denis Logunov and colleagues reported a consistent strong protective effect across all participant age groups [25]. Sputnik V vaccine is also known as Gam-COVID-Vac. It utilises adenovirus 26 (Ad26) and adenovirus 5 (Ad5) as vectors. The other two vaccines utilising the adenovirus vector approach are the Oxford–AstraZeneca vaccine, which uses a chimpanzee adenovirus (ChAdOx) [26], and the Johnson & Johnson vaccine that uses the only Ad26 [27].

Although vaccines are being evolved and clinical trials are being performed at a rapid speed, the sad part of the picture is that a lot many people who are already vaccinated have got affected by the coronavirus. Probably the mutation has caused a change in the spike of the protein which is the target area of the vaccine. Although it's a hypothetical note only as of now, if it's true, then the antibodies may not be able to recognise and neutralise the virus effectively.

Although the journey till now has remained a roller coaster ride for many, it is important to be patient and calm till the time the scientific reasons for the mutations and further effective vaccines and medicine become available. Further, people should strictly maintain hand hygiene and social distancing norms besides swearing masks all the time.

4. Lessons learnt so far

The COVID-19 pandemic has made us learn certain lessons.

1. The pandemic has reminded us of the theory proposed by Charles Darwin, which emphasised the concept of the survival of the fittest. The same concept could be applied to the COVID-19 pandemic also, as people with decreased immunity are more prone to getting COVID infection and vice versa. Hence, every possible attempt to maintain and enhance our immunity should be emphasised upon. Although there is no scientific data to suggest that a boosted immunity prevents getting COVID-19 infection, every possible effort to keep healthy and fit should be sought.

Besides, taking a healthy diet every possible attempt should be made to do physical activities like jogging, exercise, yoga, etc. Smoking and drinking should be avoided as much as possible. Junk foods should refrain.

2. No country in this world is powerful. This pandemic has made even the superpowers standstill and has shattered their economy too. Hence, it can be inferred that no country in this country is powerful. Even the smallest of the smallest nonvisible virus can be dangerous.

3. More and more trees are being cut and every effort is being made by mankind to infiltrate the wildlife sector leading to various calamities and environmental imbalance. We should thus try to maintain a balance by planting more and more trees and try to restore the imbalance being created. Thus it can be said that whatever we do we are still not beyond nature and any disturbances made within nature give reciprocating results.

4. Work can be managed from home. The exclusive usage of the digital platform during this pandemic has taught us that work can still be managed from a distant place. The development of various software are applications have made things handy. The usage of these latest technologies should further be explored and its applications should further be studied.

Furthermore, we can manage with a smaller number of vehicles. Means of travel such as subway and metros should further be developed. Emphases on cycling for small distance travel can also be propagated.

5. The pandemic has also made us realised the importance of a healthy relationship with each other and helping the persons in need. Earlier all the family members used to live together, eat, drink and leisure together. But with time with the growing social and its ever-changing rules, more and more families started moving towards nuclear family-based approach. This has led to weaker

relationships with each other. The lockdown and imposition of curfew have led family members to interact. Also, people have started helping each other in this time of need of each other.

6. The second wave seems to be the result of the casual and ignorant behaviour of the people towards the given instructions of maintaining social distancing and wearing masks. People should understand the need to maintain social distancing and hand hygiene practices. The brunt of this form of casual approach falls on people of every section of society. The second wave of the pandemic has been more devastating. Hence healthy practices like social distancing and hand wash must be regularly and strictly followed.

5. Future recommendations

1. The health care system should be revolutionised. Every effort to upgrade the health sector and strategies to tackle the pandemics should be redefined.

2. A separate front should be formulated that will take necessary urgent steps at the time of need

3. Proper allocation of places for managing affected patients should be ready beforehand.

4. Strategies for entry and exit of patients should be redefined to make minimal contact with each other

5. Guidelines for lockdown should be formulated to be crystal clear regarding the strategies to be adopted in case of any pandemic

6. Also, guidelines for the elderly and patients with immunocompromised states should be made

7. Red flag signals should be generated to timely communicate and curtail the spread of disease

8. Steps to expedite more and more speedy clinical trials should also be designed

9. As lockdown like situation affects the business domain and poor strata people majorly, upfront crucial steps should also be taken to keep the economy front balanced during the pandemic phase.

6. Conclusion

The journey through the COVID-19 pandemic has been full of major ups and downs so far.

Furthermore, though efforts are being put into the development of an effective vaccine, a big question regarding its effectiveness and side effects still prevails. Till the time effective treatment comes in the market every possible effort to maintain social distancing and hand hygiene should be practiced and followed sincerely.

Author details

Divyesh Kumar
Department of Radiotherapy and Oncology, Post Graduate Institute of Medical
Education and Research (PGIMER), Chandigarh, India

*Address all correspondence to: divyeshanand1@gmail.com

IntechOpen

References

[1] Huang C, Wang Y, Li X, Ren L, Zhao J, Hu Y, et al. Clinical features of patients infected with 2019 novel coronavirus in Wuhan, China. Lancet. 2020 Feb 15;395(10223):497-506.

[2] Cucinotta D, Vanelli M.WHO Declares COVID-19 a Pandemic. Acta Biomed.2020;91:157-160.

[3] Singhal T. A Review of Coronavirus Disease-2019 (COVID-19). Indian J Pediatr. 2020 Apr;87(4):281-286.

[4] Chaudhary M, Sodani PR, Das S. Effect of COVID-19 on Economy in India: Some Reflections for Policy and Programme. Journal of Health Management. 2020;22(2):169-180.

[5] S J, Sreedharan S. Analysing the Covid-19 Cases in Kerala: a Visual Exploratory Data Analysis Approach. SN Compr Clin Med. 2020 Aug 14:1-12.

[6] Wang D, Hu B, Hu C, Zhu F, Liu X, Zhang J, Wang B, Xiang H, Cheng Z, Xiong Y, Zhao Y, Li Y, Wang X, Peng Z. Clinical Characteristics of 138 Hospitalized Patients With 2019 Novel Coronavirus–Infected Pneumonia in Wuhan, China. JAMA. 2020 03 17;323(11):1061.

[7] Liang W, Guan W, Chen R, Wang W, Li J, Xu K, Li C, Ai Q, Lu W, Liang H, Li S, He J. Cancer patients in SARS-CoV-2 infection: a nationwide analysis in China. The Lancet Oncology. 2020 03;21(3):335-337.

[8] Finset A, Bosworth H, Butow P, Gulbrandsen P, Hulsman RL, Pieterse AH, Street R, Tschoetschel R, van Weert J. Effective health communication - a key factor in fighting the COVID-19 pandemic. Patient Educ Couns. 2020 May;103(5):873-876.

[9] Reddy B, Gupta A. Importance of effective communication during COVID-19 infodemic. J Fam Med Prim Care. 2020;9(8):3793-3796.

[10] Jena, Pravat Kumar, Impact of Pandemic COVID-19 on Education in India (July 30, 2020). International Journal of Current Research (IJCR), Vol-12, Issue-7, Page-12582-12586 (2020).

[11] Kaushal V, Srivastava S. Hospitality and tourism industry amid COVID-19 pandemic: Perspectives on challenges and learnings from India. Int J Hosp Manag. 2021 Jan;92:102707. doi: 10.1016/j.ijhm.2020.102707. Epub 2020 Oct 1. PMID: 33024348; PMCID: PMC7528873.

[12] Nhamo G, Dube K, Chikodzi D. Implications of COVID-19 on Gaming, Leisure and Entertainment Industry. Counting the Cost of COVID-19 on the Global Tourism Industry. 2020 Jul 15:273-95.

[13] United Nations Development Programme. Human development report 1994. New York: Oxford University Press; 1994.

[14] Aldis W. Health security as a public health concept: a critical analysis. Health Policy Plan. 2008;23:369-375.

[15] 15.Fukuda-Parr S. New threats to human security in the era of globalization. J Hum Dev. 2003;4: 167-179.

[16] Hardiman M. The revised International Health Regulations: a framework for global health security. Int J Antimicrob Agents. 2003;21: 207-211.

[17] Wilson K, von Tigerstrom B, McDougall C. Protecting global health security through the International Health Regulations: requirements and challenges. CMAJ. 2008;179: 44-48.

[18] Wilson K, McDougall C, Forster A. The responsibility of healthcare institutions to protect global health security. Healthc Q. 2009;12:56-60.

[19] Heymann DL, Chen L, Takemi K, Fidler DP, Tappero JW, Thomas MJ, et al. Global health security: the wider lessons from the west African Ebola virus disease epidemic. The Lancet. 2015;385(9980):1884-1901.

[20] Fragmented health systems in COVID-19: rectifying the misalignment between global health security and universal health coverage.Lal, Arush et al.The Lancet, Volume 397, Issue 10268, 61-67.

[21] 21.Garg S, Bhatnagar N, Arora E, Aggarwal P. Revisiting Global Health Security Measures in COVID 19 Pandemic. Indian J Comm Health. 2021;33(2):407-410.

[22] Scharoun K, van Caulil K, Liberman A. Bioterrorism vs. health security — crafting a plan of preparedness. Health Care Manag. 2002;21:74-92.

[23] Katz R, Singer DA. Health and security in foreign policy. Bull World Health Organ. 2007;85:233-234.

[24] Commission on Human Security. Human security now. New York: Commission on Human Security; 2003.

[25] Logunov DY Dolzhikova IV Shcheblyakov DV et al.Safety and efficacy of an rAd26 and rAd5 vector-based heterologous prime-boost COVID-19 vaccine: an interim analysis of a randomised controlled phase 3 trial in Russia.Lancet. 2021; S0140-6736(21)00234-00238.

[26] Voysey M Clemens SAC Madhi SA et al.Safety and efficacy of the ChAdOx1 nCoV-19 vaccine (AZD1222) against SARS-CoV-2: an interim analysis of four randomised controlled trials in Brazil, South Africa, and the UK.Lancet. 2021; 397: 99-111.

[27] Sadoff J Le Gars M Shukarev G et al. Safety and immunogenicity of the Ad26. COV2.S COVID-19 vaccine candidate: interim results of a phase 1/2a, double-blind, randomized, placebo-controlled trial.medRxiv. 2020; (published online Sept 25.)

Chapter 6

Time Series Forecasting on COVID-19 Data and Its Relevance to International Health Security

Steven Kraamwinkel

Abstract

The Corona virus pandemic is the most tragic virus outbreak in more than a century. Corona has globally already taken the lives of four million people, across all continents. The virus has the potential to become very catastrophic, if a significant part of the world population does not have any form of immunity against it. In this project, the aim is to make forecasts on the number of daily infections in the Netherlands. Seven different models were implemented to forecast the number of infected people in a three-month time period. The sequential CNN model outperformed all other models substantially. The capabilities of CNN models in time series forecasting can be very encouraging in conducting more research on time series data with convolutional neural networks.

Keywords: time series forecasting, data wrangling, convolutional neural network, machine learning, ARIMA, time series analysis, time series modeling, computational intelligence

1. Introduction

COVID-19 is currently a pandemic that has very serious impacts in today society. It does not only affect the health of individuals, but has also economical, social, cultural, and political consequences. Therefore is it of great importance to have Covid-19 data visible for as much possible, and to train models that are able to forecast the number of new infections on Covid-19, and to learn from them before new Covid mutations, or newer diseases occur.

The objective of this research was to make COVID-19 data more visible and interpretable, and having at least two statistical models that are able to make forecasts on COVID-19 cases using machine or deep learning techniques. It can be beneficial for future pandemics, to have models that are able to forecast and predict the possible impact a new virus can have not only on the health care sector, but on society as a whole.

Different artificial intelligence (AI) techniques can be used to aid scientists in medical and biological fields that are doing research in virology and pandemic control. And for society, more predictive analysis and data visualization that is understandable for the average person, means more awareness about past, current, and possibly future development of a virus pandemic.

1.1 The Corona virus in detail

The Corona virus, also named Covid-19, is a disease that is caused by the novel severe acute respiratory syndrome, and an infected patient shows well known symptoms such as fever, cough, and fatigue. Since the virus is able to spread via human-to-human contact from any person who is infected, the virus turned into a very catastrophic pandemic [1, 2].

The corona virus spread across the globe in less than six months from the first cases originating from the city of Wuhan in China. The World Health Organization has officially declared the corona virus as a global pandemic, and specific countries have regulated measures to reduce and overcome the severe effects of the virus.

1.2 Problem identification

The aim of this research is to implement multiple machine learning and computational intelligence (CI) models that are able to predict the number of corona infections over a certain specified time interval. In basic ML, there are two main types of learning, supervised learning and unsupervised learning. Considering the prediction of the number of corona infections in the time interval February 2021–April 2021, after observing input data from the number of infections of time interval April 2020–January 2021, the problem can be framed as a supervised learning problem. In supervised learning, an algorithm learns to make associations, also called mappings, between certain input that in many cases originates from a dataset, and certain output. Each sample originating from a dataset has an input component (x), with a corresponding output component (y). Supervised learning also aims at approximating the real underlying mapping between those inputs and outputs [3, 4].

Since the goal is to predict future values on the number of corona virus infections, the problem can also be identified as a regression type problem. This is the case, because numerical values are predicted, and given a specific input, an output in the form of a function $f : \mathbb{R}^n \rightarrow \{1, \dots \dots k\}$ is produced. Regression type problems, can be both linear and nonlinear.

1.3 Introduction to time series data and time series forecasting

Data that registers the spread and development of the corona pandemic, always takes a specific time point into account [5]. Also, all databases recording corona infections, hospitalization, and deaths always have counts of individuals taken at specific points in time. Therefore the underlying data can be considered as time series data.

Time series data can be defined as a one-dimensional time ordered sequence of values of a variable that has an attached time dependent component. It are considered measurements of any type that are observed sequentially over time or at regular time intervals [4, 6–9].

In many cases, a time series can be identified as a vector of type: $\{x^{(1)}, x^{(2)}, \dots, x^{(n)}\}$, where each element $x^{(t)} \in \mathbb{R}^m$ is an array of m values [5]. Time series data is always temporal data. This means that data is organized over time, with a time attribute being an index of the observations in the dataset [9]. Time series can be modeled in various domains, ranging from financial and stock market data, to weather and earthquake forecasting, as well as pandemics modeling and medicine intake [10].

Time series forecasting is an area of research, that is aimed at the analysis of past observations of a random variable, to develop a model that best captures underlying relationships and patterns. It contains also the prediction of future values of a random variable [1], as accurate as possible, with data that has a time component attached. All information to make any forecast is available, including historical data and knowledge of any future events that might impact the forecasts.

A typical time series forecasting model can be formulated as: $X_{t+1} = f(x_t, x_{t+1}, \ldots, x_{t-n+1})$, where x_t is the time series data. In time series data, every point x_t can be formulated by: $x_t = f_t + s_t + c_t + e_t$, which is the sum of the trend, seasonal, cyclical, and irregular components [11].

Time series forecasting can be divided into one-step forecasting, and multi-step forecasting. In one-step forecasting, the next time step is computed using the historical inputs. In multi-step forecasting, the forecast of the previous time-step is used as an input, and combined with the historical data produces the output of the next multiple time steps [4].

Forecasting is different than prediction, since forecasting considers a temporal dimension, which is always contained in any time series data. In such temporal dimension, future forecasts are always dependent on the current situation. This makes forecasting and modeling forecasts more difficult than predictive analysis [12].

Many people wrongfully assume that forecasting future values is not possible. In fact, there are computational intelligence models that can capture data patterns, and are able to make better forecasts than random guessing, and also show better performance than simple models that make average or naive forecasts. In such models, not the exact future is predicted, but it can be estimated from available real world data [13].

Time series forecasts can aid many professional in their area of work in guiding their future actions and decision making processes. For example, it can advice medical practitioners to determine the course of a treatment with a patient.

In academics, time series forecasting is considered to be one of the most profitable data mining methods, and a core skill in the data analytics field, but also a relative difficult one, and a relative unknown field of research [14–18].

The key challenge in time series datasets is the presence of time-dependent confounding variables. It is still a tremendous challenge and even an obstacle to adjust a time series model for these time-dependent confounding variables, and many forecasts made today still contain certain biases in their results [19].

2. Models for time series forecasting

Despite its relative neglect compared to other research area's in artificial intelligence, there have been numerous and also different types of models developed for time series forecasting. Two groups of models that have recently and in the past been refined for time series data are the classical machine learning models and deep learning neural networks.

2.1 Baseline models

Over the twentieth century simple and sometimes effective baseline models have been developed, that are able to make forecasts, somewhat better than random guessing. Two models that can efficiently and effectively be implemented as a baseline model in any time series modeling problem are:

- The naive model, also called a persistence model. A model that uses the last seen observation as the forecast [20], and assumes that all future values are equal to the last observed point [21].

- The simple average model, which uses as the forecasting value, the average value over all previously observed input values [4].

2.2 Classical machine learning models

Classical machine learning models also named statistical models, were originally developed from the 1960's and later decades for predictive analysis. These models use the variables historical past to predict future observations [9], and are linear. Some of these methods, like ARIMA and Exponential Smoothing, are still widely used. This is mainly because of their high accuracy, robustness, efficiency, and the fact that they can be used by non-experts in machine learning [22]. Most of these methods make use of a concept called lagged prediction. This means that for a prediction of time t, it relies on t-1 and so on, all the way until t-n. In other words, it relies on data points that are in the previous period of time [23].

2.2.1 Auto regressive model

A statistical model where the value of interest is forecasted using a linear combination of past values of the variable, is called an autoregressive model [24]. Autoregression is a term that indicates that the predicted values are a regression of the current value of that variable against one or more prior values. The autoregressive (AR(p)) model is a stochastic model, that assumes some form of randomness in data. This means that future forecasts can be made with high accuracy, but not very close to being 100% accurate [9].

These models were developed from the concept that models are developed by regressing on previous values, also called lag terms [19]. An autoregressive model (AR(p)) can be formulated by:

$$y_t = c + \phi_1 y_1 - 1 + \phi_2 y_t - 2 + \; ... \; + \phi_n y_t - p + \epsilon_t \tag{1}$$

where ϵ_t is white noise or error term, and $\phi_{1, ... \; ... \; ...}, \; \phi_n$ are parameters [6, 7].

2.2.2 Moving average model

A moving average model is a model based on error lag regression. It is a stochastic process whose output values are linearly dependent on the weighted sum of a white noise error and the error term from previous time values [19, 20, 24].

A moving average model (MA(q)), builds a function of error terms of the past [11], and is basically the weighted sum of the current and past random errors [9]. A first order MA(q) model can be expressed by:

$$y_t = c + \epsilon_t + \theta_1 \epsilon_{t-1} \tag{2}$$

A higher-order MA(q) model can be expressed by the following formula:

$$y_t = c + \epsilon_t + \theta_1 \epsilon_{t-1} + \theta_2 \epsilon_{t-2} + \theta_q \epsilon_{t-q} \tag{3}$$

2.2.3 ARIMA

A very popular and in many situations also an effective model in time series forecasting, is the ARIMA model, which is the acronym for AutoRegresive Integrated MovingAverage model. ARIMA models combine the AR and MA models, with an integrated (I-part) to an ARIMA model, that can make any data stationary by means of differencing [11, 24]. The model was orginally developed by the famous statisticians Box and Jenkins in 1968.

The purpose of an ARIMA model is to describe autocorrelations in time series data [6, 21].

An ARIMA model is a typical linear model, that assumes a linear correlation between the time-series values. It makes use of these linear dependencies to extract local patterns, and removes high-frequency noise from the underlying data [1, 16, 25].

ARIMA models have proven to be very accurate forecasting models for short-term forecasting, when there is a scarcity of trainable data [26]. It is arguably one of the most popular and widely used linear models in time series forecasting, due to its great flexibility and performance [16].

Any ARIMA model has three main hyperparameters; p, d, and q. The p parameter stands for the number of lag observations, the d parameter defines the degree of differencing, and the q parameter describes the previous error terms used to predict the future value [8, 9, 20, 26, 27].

The values for the p, d, and q values can be determined after plotting the ACF and PACF plot. ARIMA models are relatively simple to construct, and often show better performance that more complex, structural models [28].

Eq. (4) below shows the mathematical ARIMA model, in the following formula:

$$X_t = \alpha + \beta_1 X_{t-1} + \beta_2 X_{t-2} + \ ...\ + \beta_p X_{t-p} + \theta_1 \epsilon_{t-1} + \theta_2 \epsilon_{t-2} + \ ...\ + \theta_q \epsilon_{t-q} \qquad (4)$$

where α is the intercept term, $\beta_1 \ ...\ ..\ \beta_p$ are lag coefficients, $\theta_1 \ ...\ ...\ \theta_q$ are the moving average coefficients, and $\epsilon_{t-1} ... \epsilon_{t-q}$ are errors.

2.2.4 Exponential smoothing

Exponential smoothing (ES) models are based on a description of trend and seasonality in the data, and the prediction is a weighted linear sum of recent past observations or lags [24]. In single exponential smoothing, there is a parameter α, the smoothing factor, which is an exponentially decreasing weight decay factor of past observations [1, 4, 6, 7]. Exponential smoothing can be formulated and computed as follows:

$$s_t = \alpha x_t + (1 - \alpha) s_{t-1} = s_{t-1} + \alpha(x_t - s_{t-1}) \qquad (5)$$

where $t > 0$, and where $t > 0$, and α is the smoothing factor, which can be set at any number ranging between 0 and 1 [23].

This means that for predictive purposes, the more recent observations have more weight in the computed predicted values, than the observations further away in the past [29]. Especially when the smoothing factor, α has a higher value close to 1. Any smoothing method on time series data will oftentimes yield sufficient performance with univariate data that contains low trend or seasonality [24]. It also requires only a low amount of computation power [23].

2.2.5 Holt-winters exponential smoothing

Holt-Winters exponential smoothing is also called triple exponential smoothing. It is a smoothing method that is similar to exponential smoothing models, where the next time step is an exponentially weighted linear function of observations at prior time steps. It is a more advanced smoothing method, since it also takes trend and seasonality into account when making forecasts. Therefore, HWES is suitable for univariate time series with trend and also seasonal components [24], and often performs well.

2.3 Time series forecasting with neural networks

A neural network can be thought of as a network of neurons which are organized in layers, weights that are added to some of the networks parameters, and an activation function that causes the network to converge towards minimizing or maximizing an objective [30].

An artificial neural network (ANN) has a data-driven approach, where training depends on the available data. Furthermore, ANN models do not make any assumptions about the statistical distribution of the underlying time series, and are able to perform consistently non-linear modeling [20].

The goal of any ANN is to optimize an algorithm towards an objective function. This optimization is the process of finding optimal values for parameters or function arguments that minimizes or maximizes that function [3].

ANN's are flexible and non-parametric methods, which can perform nonlinear mappings from data. They are able, similar to other machine learning methods, to generalize over data. This is a process called generalization, and is the ability of a machine learning algorithm to perform well on new and previously unseen inputs. The generalization error, also mentioned as the test error, is the expected value of the error on a new input. It can be estimated by measuring its performance on a test set of examples that were collected separately from the training set, by performance metrics. In the research the two performance metrics are the root mean squared error (RMSE), and the mean average error (MAE) [3].

Neural networks are stochastic by nature. This means that given the same model configuration and the same training set, a different internal set of weights will result each time the model is trained to a different performance [4].

Today, deep learning is centered around artificial neural networks, than can be defined as a non linear function from a set of input variables x to a set of output variables y, controlled by a vector w of adjustable parameters. These networks allow nonlinear relationships between the response variable and its predictors, and are able to overcome the challenges faced by linear statistical models [6, 20].

A typical neural network always contains an activation function, an optimization procedure, and a set of hyperparameters. Many different functions can serve as an activation function, because a neural network is able to approximate any continuous function that maps input values to output values [30]. Most commonly used activation functions are the Sigmoid, ReLu, LeakyReLu, Tanh, and Softmax functions. In the network during the optimization procedure, an optimization algorithm makes the network converge towards the best optimal solution, which is minimizing or maximizing the objective. This can be considered as finding the appropriate values of parameters $\theta_1...\theta_n$ [6, 31].

Parameters are in any ANN the weights for each variable or feature in the ANN model. In many cases they are determined by the backpropagation algorithm and iterations made by the optimizing function [32]. Hyperparameters in a neural network are settings whose values can be determined and manually modified from outside the algorithm itself, and that controls the capacity of a model [3, 32].

2.3.1 ANN learning process

The learning process of an ANN consists of modeling past observations with the objective of estimating the underlying temporal relationships [25]. Any artificial neural network learns by a procedure called the backpropagation procedure. In an artificial neural network the backpropagation procedure make the network learn and update its parameters after each training epoch. In detail, it evaluates the gradient of an error function by backpropagating the errors backwards through the network. The resulting derivatives are than used to compute new values for the neural networks weights. These adjustments can lead to significant improvements in optimization of the objective error function, and aim to minimize the error function [5, 30, 33].

In deep learning solutions, when a model converges to a local minimum, that result is accepted, since the loss function is approximately minimized [3]. This characteristic makes any artificial neural network as an approximator to any objective.

Most deep learning optimization algorithms are based on the stochastic gradient descent algorithm. SGD is an optimization algorithm that aims to maximize or minimize an objective function, in this research an error function, also called a loss function [3].

When the algorithm operates on a training set of examples, it usually follows the estimated gradient downhill towards a local or global minimum, that optimizes any objective function [3, 30].

In the predictions produced by a neural network there is always an element of randomness. Therefore the network is trained multiple times where each training cycle is called an epoch. An epoch can be defined as a pass through the training set, where a pass includes both a forward and a backward pass through the neural network. The number of epochs denotes how many passes, forward and backward, were required for the best training of the model. During one epoch the neural network with all the training data is trained for one cycle [22, 34]. After a fixed number of epochs, training of the network stops, and the average or best result of all epochs becomes the resulting output of the neural network [6].

In the time series forecasting domain different deep learning models can be applied. The most commonly used deep learning models in time series forecasting are: the multi-layer perceptron (MLP), the recurrent neural network (RNN), and the convolutional neural network (CNN) [31]. For this regression type problem, RNN and CNN networks are promising solutions [10].

2.3.2 MultiLayer perceptron

A multilayer perceptron is a relatively simple artificial neural network that is used to approximate a mapping function from input variables to output variables. The network is more commonly known as a "feedforward neural network". It can be applied as a deep learning model to any time series forecasting, since the network is robust to noise from the input data. It does not make strong assumptions about the mapping function, and is capable to learn complex and high-dimensional mappings, and both linear and nonlinear relationships [35]. MLP's are memory-less, are unidirectional where neurons are grouped in two or more layers [36], and use the feed forward neural network architecture with backpropagation [20]. The neural network aims to generalize over data samples, such that newer samples are produced beyond by what is known by the model itself. It can therefore make accurate and valuable forecasts.

One key limitation is that a MLP has to specify the temporal dependence upfront during the design of the model [4].

2.3.3 Recurrent neural networks

Recurrent neural networks are a type of ANN with the following characteristics:

- RNN's have typically been used in the modeling of sequences, and were developed for modeling data with a time dimension [17, 19], and are capable of modeling seasonal patterns [22].

- RNN's can automatically learn the temporal dependence and correlations from data [2]. Considering this temporal dependence for past observations have been proven to a successful methodology for time series forecasting [26].

- One observation at a time can be shown from a sequence, and the model can learn what observations it has seen previously that are relevant and how they are relevant to the forecasting [4].

In the RNN model architecture, both a mapping from inputs to outputs, and the context from the input sequence useful for the mapping are learned [4]. Each RNN cell contains an internal memory state that serves as a summary of past information, and it is repeatedly updated with new observations for every time step [19].

Besides its overall better performance, flexibility, and improved memory capabilities compared to the MLP, RNN's are computationally more expensive. The overall process takes significant computation time [10, 17]. Also, standard RNN's have difficulty in learning long-term dependencies [26], and could make poor forecasts because of the vanishing gradient problem in larger sequences. This means that RNN's are not capable of carrying long-term dependencies [5, 22].

There are two specific variants of the recurrent neural network, namely the long short term memory (LSTM), and the gated recurrent unit (GRU) networks [22].

A LSTM network model has special LSTM units that are composed of cells, where each has an input gate, output gate, and a forget gate [31]. The input gate and forget gate determine how much of the past information is retained in the current cell state for each LSTM cell, and also how much of the current information to propagate forward [22].

The model learns a function that maps a sequence of past observations as input to an output observation. It reads one time step of the sequence at a time and builds up an internal state representation that can be used as a learned context for making predictions [4]. It is a special RNN variant, since the model is able to learn long term dependencies [8, 22], by replacing the hidden layers of a RNN with memory cells. Each cell in the LSTM network remembers the desired values over arbitrary time intervals [31]. Furthermore, it is able to overcome to most common limitation of standard RNN's, the vanishing gradient problem [2, 10, 19, 26].

Another RNN variant is the Gated Recurrent Unit (GRU), which is recently developed, first in 2014. It is an artificial neural network that uses an input gate, forget gate, update gate, and reset gate. Each gate is a vector, that decides what information should be passed to the output gate. The update gate decides how much of the last memory to keep. The reset gate defines how to combine the new input with the previous memory [8]. The GRU on average is not the most successful model in forecasting, but is less complicated to build and computations made by a GRU are faster than the LSTM. Also, it often shows competitive performances compared to ARIMA and RNN models.

2.3.4 Convolutional neural network

A convolutional neural network (CNN) is a specialized kind of neural network for processing data that has a known grid-like topology. It is different from other known neural networks since it uses convolutions instead of matrix multiplications in at least one layer. The input of a convolutional matrix can be a matrix, or a sequence. Also typical CNN's do not need medium of large sized datasets to perform excellent, only require a small set of parameters, and are able to make connection when data is sparse. Time series data can be considered as a type of 1-D grid taking samples at regular time intervals [3].

A convolutional neural network combines three architectural ideas; local receptive fields, shared weights, and spatial or temporal subsampling [35]. In a CNN, a sequence of observations can be treated like a one-dimensional(1-D) image, what a CNN can read and distill the most pertinent elements. In a 1-D CNN, the network uses inputs within its local receptive field to make forecasts [19]. CNN's support both univariate and multivariate input data and supports efficient feature learning [4].

Layers in a typical CNN model are the convolutional layer, the hidden layer, a pooling layer, a flatten layer, and a dense layer [4]. The convolutional layer has to ability to extract useful knowledge. The pooling layer distills and sub samples the output of the convolutional layer to the most salient elements [10], it thereby reduces the size of the convolved feature, in this research the input sequence. A flatten layer is implemented as a layer between the convolutional and dense layer to reduce the feature maps to a single one-dimensional vector. And the dense layer is a fully connected layer, similar to an MLP, which at a final stage of the CNN network, interprets the features extracted by the convolutional part of the model [3, 37]. **Figure 1** illustrates the one dimensional sequential CNN architecture, and how any input data is transformed by the convolutional operations into certain output.

A convolutional neural network has a kernel, that can be considered as a tiny window. The kernel slides over the input sequence or matrix, and applies the convolution operation on each subregion, called a patch, that the kernel meets across the input data. It functions as a filer that extracts the features from any 1-D sequence or higher dimensional image. This results in a convolved matrix, which is more useful than the original features of the input data, and often improves modeling performance [10].

In training a convolutional network, a forward pass executes training on the entire network, from the initial layer to the final dense layer. Loss is calculated and during the backward pass, in a the backpropagation procedure. This procedure takes place by computing local gradients for each CNN gate: δ output/δ input for each input/output

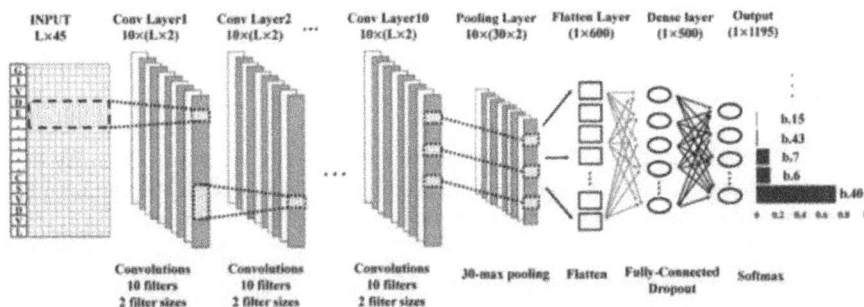

Figure 1.
1-D sequential CNN model architecture.

combination, also with use of convolutions. Similar as in the forward phase, one matrix slides over the other, what results in the computation of a local gradient. These local gradients are found and than taken together with the use of the chain rule that completely propagates all the gradients back through the convolutional network [38]. Afterwards, the networks parameters in each layer are updated [37].

A CNN can be very effective at automatically extracting and learning features from one-dimensional sequence data, such as univariate time series data, and can directly output a in multi-step vector [4]. Also, pooling operations in the neural network can significantly reduce the number of required network parameters, and makes the model more robust [10]. This can result in faster training and less overfitting on training data [37].

2.4 Automatic machine learning

Automatic machine learning (AutoML) is a research area in the AI field that focuses on the automatic optimization of ML and CI hyperparameters, stages and pipelines [39]. This results in the further development of function methods that allows complex data preparation, feature extraction, and CI modeling in fewer lines of code without the need of building whole machine learning and data science frameworks from scratch [32].

It therefore becomes easier for novices in machine learning to build competitive models, and for machine learning experts in building complex models faster [29]. This is because two main barriers, structured programming and higher mathematics, are bypassed with the progressions made by AutoML. Examples of application of AutoML that are used in this research are hyperparameter tuning in the ARIMA model, and feature engineering in the pre modeling phase.

3. Methodology

The objective of time series forecasting is the development of one or more mathematical or advanced deep learning models, that can explain the observed behavior of a time series, and possibly forecast future states of the series.

The actual time series research was subdivided into the following tasks:

- Exploratory data analysis.

- Data wrangling.

- Analysis of the time series.

- Model construction and implementation.

3.1 Exploratory data analysis

Exploratory data analysis can be considered as the set of techniques that try to maximize insight into the data, uncover the underlying structure of the data, and the extraction of important variables and features [7]. For time series analysis, to understand the underlying data and its characteristics, plotting the data is very useful. When plotting time series data, there are always two variables; the time scale on the x-axis, and the numerical variable on the y-axis. Most commonly used plots in time series data analysis are; run sequence plots, lag plots, autocorrelation plots, partial autocorrelation plots, histograms, and box plots. These time series plots can determine what models would be appropriate to model the time series.

3.1.1 Run sequence plot

The run sequence plot is in time series analysis another name for the line plot. It shows the development of the corona virus infections over time in line graph format. In this particular plot, the 7-day moving average per day is also included. **Figure 2** shows the development of the number of COVID-19 cases over a time period april 2020 - april 2021.

3.1.2 Lag plot

A lag plot can check for randomness in data. If data is random than the data should not show any identifiable structure in the lag plot, such as linearity [7]. Plotting a lag plot can be very efficient, since it quickly concludes if time series data is random or not. If such data is not random, than a random walk model for forecasting would not be appropriate.

3.1.3 Auto correlation and partial auto correlation plot

From every collection of time series data samples, its auto correlation is its most important internal structure to analyze, besides trend and seasonality.

The auto correlation function (ACF) shows how similar the previous term and the current term are. In fact, autocorrelation shows the correlation coefficients between current and previous values [9].

Autocorrelation can be defined as the second order moment $E(x_p x_{\{t + h\}} = g(h)$, that is a function of only the time lag h, and independent of the actual time index t.

It measures the degree of linear dependency between the time series at index t, and the time series at indices t-h or t + h. A positive auto correlation indicates that the present and future values of the time series move in the same direction. A negative auto correlation illustrates present and future values moving in the opposite direction [40]. If a ACF is close to 1, there is an upward trend, and an increasing value in the time series is often followed by another increase. Also, when the ACF is negative and close to −1, a decrease will probably be followed by another decrease [9].

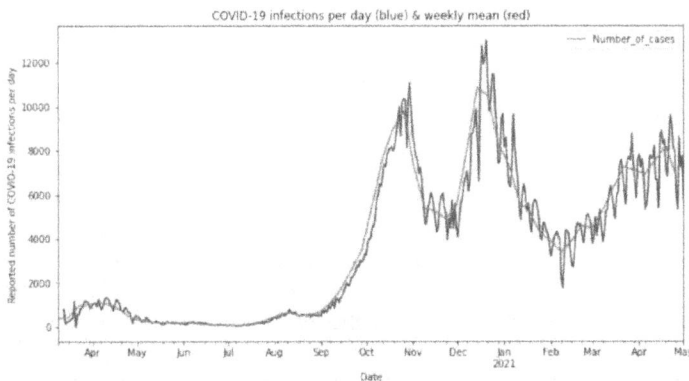

Figure 2.
Run sequence plot of the number of corona infections per day.

The auto correlation function is used to determine if the time series data is stationary of non-stationary. The function can be plotted into a graph, a correlogram, called the ACF plot, which is a plot of the autocorrelation of a time series by its lag. It is used in the model identification stage for various Box-Jenkins (ARIMA) models. If the data is truly stationary, the ACF plot will drop to zero very quickly after a few lags, while a the line graph in the ACF plot of any non-stationary data will converge to zero very slowly.

A partial autocorrelation function (PACF) in time series analysis defines the correlation between x_t and $x_{\{t + h\}}$, that is not accounted for by lags t + 1 and t + h-1. It actually measures the correlation between the time series with a lagged version of itself, but after eliminating the variations already explained by the intervening comparisons [18].

The ACF and PACF plots can tell if an autoregressive (AR) or moving average (MA) model, or both, can be appropriate. If the ACF plot shows a few serious spikes in the beginning, but not in later lags, than its recommended to model the time series data with an AR model, and use the AR component (p > 0) in the ARIMA model. If the PACF plot shows serious data spikes in the beginning, and in later lags, but only very few spikes in the ACF plot, than it is recommended to use the MA model, and make use of the MA component (q > 0) in the ARIMA model. If cases when both charts show many significances, it is recommended to model the data with an autoregressive moving average (ARMA) or autoregressive integrated moving average (ARIMA) model [40].

ACF and PACF plots are also useful for hyperparameter tuning ARIMA models, and both plot can indicate upper and lower bound values in the grid search for the p and q parameters [40].

3.1.4 Other plots

Other visualization plots that can be used to understand the time series data, are commonly used dataplots in statistics such as the QQ-plot, histogram and boxplot.

A QQ-plot helps to determine whether or not datapoints are normally distributed [9, 11]. A histogram represents the distribution of numerical data, and shows the shape of the variables distribution. The boxplot will display how data is distributed, based on minimum value, first quartile, median, third quartile, and maximum value. The smaller the boxplot, the less variability in data values [41]. These plots can be easily plotted in with Pythons matplotlib and seaborn libraries.

3.2 Data wrangling

The data wrangling process applied in this research contains data pre-processing techniques such as data preparation, feature selection, feature engineering, and data aggregation.

Data pre-processing is an important, but also time consuming process in the field of data science, which has gained importance over the past decade. This is because most CI algorithms have not been made for time series data [42].

Also, most CI models rely on high quality data in order to improve modeling performance from models that operate in real-world environments [43]. Thus, to effectively run a model and yield results, pre-processing of real-time and time series data is necessary.

In any large dataset only the most relevant features are selected, and irrelevant information, what does not have any influence on the desired output, is removed in a data pre-processing process called feature subset selection. This leads consequently to dimensionality reduction in data, and having a learning algorithms that operates faster and more effective on more simple input data [41].

Also feature engineering and data aggregation are applied, since the cumulative values from the original dataset are transformed into its single original date values, by means of differencing, groupby mechanisms, and resampling data to daily sums. This creates new features to day scale, which make the Covid-19 data more suitable for analytical and modeling purposes [32, 39, 44].

Also these data transformation techniques are able to reduce noise in the time series data, and produce smoothing of the original time series [11].

For example, in the run sequence plots, a 7-day moving average calculated over the daily sum is plotted, which has a smoothing effect on the data, in the same plot as the daily sums. This is a statistic that is computed by sliding a window, in this research seven days, over the daily series, that aggregates the data for every window [11].

In the later modeling stage, data from the used dataset will be divided in a smaller data subset, by a process called instance reduction [43]. For modeling simplicity, only months that contains data from every day of the month are considered. Since the used dataset starts recording the Corona virus infections from 13 March 2020, March 2020 is not included in the used data. The input data for every models contains the number of corona virus infections, from April 2020 until and including April 2021.

3.3 Time series analysis

Time series data can be considered as a series of measurements, or a sequence of observations that are indexed in time order [45]. An important aspect in time series is fitting models on historical data, and using these model to predict future observations.

Not every chunk of data can be considered and treated in similar ways. Data is only considered as time series data when it has a datetime measurement, also called a time component. This makes the time series data different from other types of data, but also more difficult to interpret. Time series data adds specifically a time dimension, which means an explicit order dependence between observations. In these instances, each data point in a time series depends on previous data points from that same time series [13].

Time series analysis is about the use of statistical methods and machine learning algorithms to extract certain information and characteristics of data, in order to predict future values based on stored past time series data [23]. Time series analysis is different than other analysis in supervised machine learning. Time series cannot be considered as a standard linear regression problem, since the assumption that observations are independent does not hold [6]. In the case of time series data, each data value depends on the previous data value, and is so called lag dependent. Therefore time series analysis cannot be solved with simple linear regression.

Time series analysis is the phase in the whole time series process that follows right after the exploratory data analysis. In any time series analysis data plot, the x-axis has in many cases the time variable, showing the amount of a numerical variable plotted on the y-axis at specific datetime points and time interval [46].

Time series data can be univariate or multivariate. Univariate time series data are datasets containing a single series of observations with a temporal ordering and a model is required to learn a function from the series of past observations to predict one or more new output values. In multivariate time series data there is more than one variable observed at each time step [4, 15].

3.3.1 Stationarity

One very important characteristic for time series data, is that the data needs to be stationary before doing any forecasts in many classical ML models. Time series data that are "stationary" have values that fluctuate around a constant mean or have a constant variance, that does not change over time [11, 28]. This means that a change it time, for example taking the time series of a newer year or month, does not change the shape of the distribution when all data is stationary [9]. Also, stationary time series have no predictable pattern in the long-term [23].

Non-stationarity is in many cases caused by fluctuations in trend or seasonality [6, 7]. When the data is non-stationary, it can be set stationary with differencing, or with a method called time series decomposition [11, 15].

3.3.2 Differencing

Any time series can be made stationary with first-order or higher-order differencing [20]. It transforms the data in a way that a previous observation is subtracted from the current observation, and thereby removes any trend and seasonality structure of the time series data [18, 23].

The differencing approach is used as one of the main parameters in the Box-Jenkins ARIMA model [45]. First order differencing is mathematically formulated by: $d = 1$, $x_t = x_t - x_{\{t-1\}}$, and second order differencing by: $d = 2$, $x_t = x_t - 2x_{\{t-1\}} - x_{\{t-2\}}$ [11].

In this research, first order differencing is applied, and can be easily computed with the python. diff() build-in function.

3.3.3 Time series decomposition

Data can often consist of multiple patterns, and can show linear or cyclic behavior. Therefore data splitting into multiple components can be very beneficial to improve understanding, and to discover any irregularities or white noise. The process of splitting or dividing time series data into multiple components is called time series decomposition [18].

Any time series model can be decomposed in trend, seasonality, and irregular components. The trend component is the pattern and behavior of the data in the long term. It is a certain pattern of growth of the data, and a description of the variable over a certain period of time. The seasonal component is a particular pattern in the time series data, that is repeated at specific time periods. Irregular components can be considered as data that is far off-trend. It contains abnormal values, sometimes called residual or outliers. It is also referred to as "white noise". Time series data can also contain cyclical components. These can be considered as movements observed after every few units of time, but they occur less frequently than seasonal fluctuations [11].

The objective of time series decomposition is to model the long-term trend and seasonality, and to estimate the overall time series as a combination of them [11]. A time series decomposition model can be additive or multiplicative. When the time series data appears to have any sort of changing seasonality pattern, the multiplicative decomposition model is recommended, in other cases the additive model is endorsed [7].

3.3.4 Augmented dickey fuller test

The augmented dickey fuller (ADF) test is a statistical unit root test that is used to determine stationarity of a time series, and the magnitude of the trend component

[8, 11]. It is a hypothesis test, and any time series can be considered as stationary(where H_0 is false), with 95% confidentiality, when the ADF's p-value is less than 0.05 [18].

The ADF unit root test should at first be applied on the original time series that has not been differenced, to check if the data is already stationary. If not, than data should be stationarized with first order or higher order differencing [11, 15, 20].

3.3.5 Smoothing with moving averaging

Smoothing can be defined as the removal of noise from data, and can be applied in both regression and clustering problems [44]. In time series data, smoothing can be applied as a rolling moving average over a number time steps [18]. In this cases a one week(7-day) or one month(30-day) moving average can be computed. For each day, the moving average changes, since the method makes use of the sliding window, taking the average over different days [21].

Smoothing is also applied as a modeling technique that assigns weights to observations, whereas the most recent observations have more weight, than observation further away in the past. Examples of these techniques are single exponential smoothing, and triple(Holt-Winters) exponential smoothing.

3.4 Model construction and implementation

The final objective of time series analysis is the development of one or more mathematical or advanced deep learning models, that can explain the observed behavior of a time series, and possibly forecast future states of the series.

The construction and implementation of multiple time series forecasting models can be divided into the following parts:

- Data preprocessing.

- Data plotting.

- Model building.

- Model evaluation.

- Model improvement.

One of the first steps in performing time series research is to determine what data will be used for training a computational intelligence model, and what data will be used to test the performance of that model. The input sequence is divided into a training set and a test set. The sequence contains thirteen months of data, measured and aggregated to a total of 395 observations, where each observation is one day. Of those 395 days, 306 days are taken as the training set, the remaining 89 days are the test set. For the total time series data, around 77.5% is used as training data, and approximately 22.5% as testing data.

3.4.1 Data pre-processing and data plotting

Before data is used as input for a CI model, is it pre-processed first. For the dataset, only the most relevant features are selected in a process called feature selection. Secondly, all relevant data is transformed into its shape that is useful for modeling with data aggregation, which contains rescaling and resampling the time series data.

Before data gets fed to a CI model, the data is plotted to recognize its underlying structure, to determine what models can be suitable to model the time series data. In the classical time series models, the run sequence plot is plotted with a seven day moving average applied as a method for smoothing the data. The ARIMA model contains multiple data plots in its pre modeling phase, including the run sequence plot, lag plot, QQ plot, ACF plot, and PACF plot. Before constructing the CNN, it is very beneficial to have sufficient understanding in the underlying data patterns. Therefore, before building the CNN model, the data was plotted and interpreted with run sequence, ACF, and first-order differences plots.

3.4.2 Model building

Since the input time series data is univariate, and contains one column, it is best practice to extract the whole time series and store it in a variable [9].

The baseline model that is constructed in this research, simply calculates the average of all the training examples, and takes that average as its forecast.

Any AR model can be defined by an ARIMA(x, 0, 0), where x is the autoregressive parameter, a positive integer ranging between 1 and 5. The MA model is defined by an ARIMA(0, 0, x), where x is the moving average parameter, what is also a positive integer, that in many cases ranges between 1 and 5. In the ARIMA model, all three parameters from the ARIMA(p, d, q) model needs to be defined, including the differencing parameter d, because the data is non-stationary. In both exponential smoothing models, the smoothing factor needs to be determined by manual input. An optimal search would be to run a smoothing model twice, on a smoothing factor of 0.1 and 0.9, and check the performance metrics. Than can be determined if the smoothing factor needs have a high value close to 1, or a low value close to 0.

In the CNN model, the training and testing data can be split with the split_sequence function. After reshaping the input data, all CNN operations transform the sequence into a 1-D output vector. The model is fitting and best predictions are made after performing two thousand epoch training cycles.

When running and testing any model, it is run against the testing set to predict data it has not seen before.

3.4.3 Model evaluation

To evaluate a models performance, first some intuition from its characteristics is required, before making any judgments. This can be done with summarizing or describing its outcomes.

The baseline model is summarized with the .describe() function. It is a function that gives the count, mean, standard deviation, and all the boxplot values [11].

All other model are summarized with the .summarize() function.

The essential aspect in model evaluation is determining how well its forecasting results are. Performance measures such as the (root) mean squared error are a way of measuring the performance of a model [1, 3]. The following two performance measures determine the effectiveness of each model:

- Root mean squared error (RMSE). Measures the square root of the average of the squared errors of each data value [9]. It has the effect that large forecasting errors significantly increase the RMSE performance metric.

- Mean absolute error (MAE). Is the average of the forecast error values, and forces all error values to be positive [47].

3.4.4 Model improvement

When a model is performing less accurate than expected, the model can be improved. The modeling improvement step is however not a mandatory step, and is only needed when a model performs poorly than was originally intended.

In any AR, MA, ARMA, and ARIMA model, the modeling performances can be improved with hyperparameter tuning. It is considered as important in CI, since it evaluates the model to be implemented on different configurations, in order to find the best set of hyperparameters that yields in the best predictive performance [39].

Grid search is a search method that can do any hyperparameter tuning. It is a brute-force and semi-automatic based search method that explores all possible model configurations within a user specified parameter range, and is considered as an exhaustive search that often takes relatively long runtime [22, 39].

One important metric that is used in tuning hyperparameters, is the Akaike Information Criterion (AIC). It measures the relative quality of the model being considered for the description of the phenomenon, and is proven to be fast and efficient. Its value shows an estimate of the information lost, when a specific order of the model is being considered. The smaller the value of the AIC, the less information is lost, and the more accurate the model is considered to be [9].

4. Used models

4.1 Baseline model

The research started with the setup of a simple and consistent baseline model. The purpose of a baseline model is out of simplicity and for setting the boundaries for all the other models. It also helps understanding the data better, and could determine whether or not more data preparation or feature engineering is necessary [48]. If a more complex model performs worse than the baseline model, it can be considered as a poor model for forecasting the specific dataset.

The simple average model discussed in the previous section, serves in this research as the baseline model. A simple average can be implemented with formula [21]:

$$\hat{y}_{t+1} = \frac{1}{x} \sum_{i=1}^{t} y_i \qquad (6)$$

Most baseline models serve as a benchmark in forecasting research for comparing new methods to this simple method [6].

Since pandemic infections have the tendency to suddenly increase, but also to decrease very quickly in some cases, a naive or persistence model, that predicts the last seen value, would not be a model to consider as a baseline model.

4.2 Classical machine learning models

The classical machine learning, or statistical models that are implemented assume that observations are continuous, time is discrete and equally spaced, and that there are no missing observations [28].

The classical machine learning methods that are implemented are the moving average and autoregressive models, the simple exponential smoothing model, and the triple (Holt-Winters) exponential smoothing model. Special focus in the research in spend on modeling the ARIMA model, since ARIMA is a very popular and quite accurate model in time series forecasting.

4.3 CNN model

In this research one promising neural network will be implemented and tested on the COVID-19 data, the convolutional neural network (CNN) model. The CNN network that is implemented in this research, treats the input data as a sequence over which convolutional read operations can be performed, in a similar fashion as in one dimensional images [49].

The CNN model is a univariate multi-step one-dimensional vector output forecasting model. Univariate, means that one feature will be forecasted, and multi step defines the output of a sequence with multiple output values.

The CNN architecture includes an activation function, and an optimization algorithm. The activation function used in the convolutional neural network, is the ReLu activation function. It is a function that is able to overcome the problem of exploding and vanishing gradients, which occur in typical ANN's like the MLP and RNN [4]. It can be defined as ReLU = R(z) = max(0,z) [31, 32]. When activating, negative and zero inputs will have zero output, and positive inputs will be exactly the same. The ReLU activation function, therefore consistently filters out negative numbers [50].

The optimization function that is used in the CNN model, is the ADAM algorithm, which is a modified version of the SGD algorithm, and an adaptive learning rate optimization algorithm. It uses running averages and both the gradients and second moments of the gradients [31]. It has a built-in tensorflow implementation, and requires the learning rate parameter to operate [22]. The learning rate, in many cases denoted as α, indicates at which pace the weights in the neural network get updated [32]. It is currently the most commonly used optimization algorithm in artificial neural networks [3, 51].

4.4 Python packages

The research conducted in the classical statistical models rely on a few well known and frequently applied Python-packages, such as Pandas, Numpy, and Matplotlib. The Seaborn libary is used for some data visualizations. For specific time series analysis the python library Statsmodels is often used. It is a Python package that includes basic tools and models for time series analysis and modeling, and is specifically build for time series data [43]. It also provides all functionality required to model an ARIMA and exponential smoothing model [26].

Another package that is applied is pmdarima, which is used in the hyperparameter tuning of the ARIMA model [14, 52].

Sklearn, a famous python library in machine learning, is used for evaluating performance metrics of all trained CI models [43].

In the modeling phase of the 1-D sequential CNN model, the Keras library performs all CNN operations. Keras is a python library that is extensively used in many deep learning modeling situations.

5. Research results

In the time series analysis results, the lag plot as displayed in **Figure 3** indicates that the data containing the daily COVID-19 cases is non-random. Since the plot

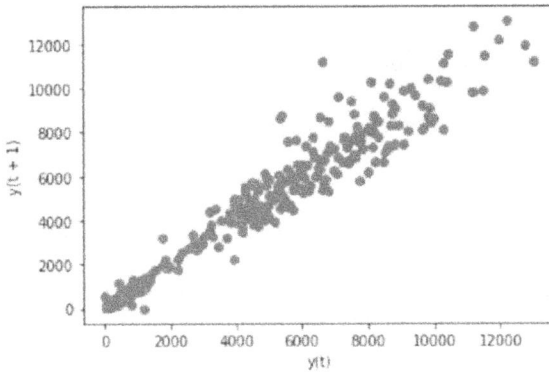

Figure 3.
Lag plot of the number of corona infections per day.

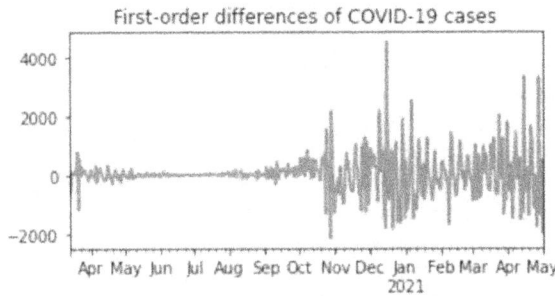

Figure 4.
First order differences number of Covid-19 infections.

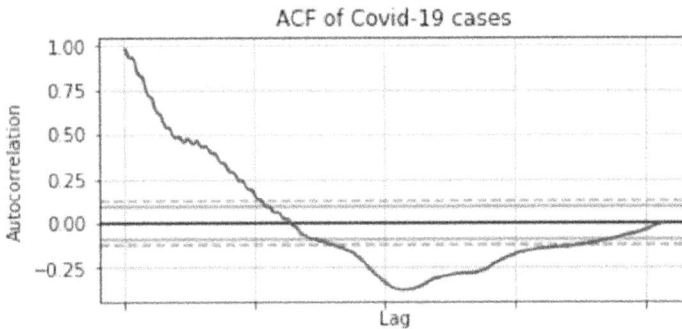

Figure 5.
ACF plot of the number of Covid-19 infections.

clearly shows a linear structure between y(t) and its lag y(t + 1), the data can be considered as non-random and suitable for time series forecasting.

First order differences as displayed in **Figure 4** show the daily changes, and clearly indicates upward and downward trends in the data starting from October 2020, up and until April 2021. **Figure 5** shows the autocorrelation function of the data of the first 400 lags. The ACF graph slowly moves to the zero value, indicating that the data is non-stationary. Therefore, differencing and appling an ARIMA model with the differencing paramater set at a value of at least 1, is strongly advised.

Model name	RMSE score	MAE score
Simple Average (SA) – Baseline model	3222.91	2733.16
Autotregressive (AR)	2913.90	2369.61
Moving average (MA)	3224.08	2736.03
Exponential smoothing (ES)	1817.11	1567.40
Holt-Winters ES (HWES)	1611.34	1379.34
ARIMA	2172.88	1721.42
1-D sequential CNN	**409.86**	**315.99**

Table 1.
Performance of all seven implemented models.

In the modeling phase, all models have been constructed, implemented, and have produced forecasts in the Jupyter notebook environment, in python 3 code. Each forecast made by each of the seven models was measured against the test set, and resulted into a root mean-squared error (RMSE) and mean average error (MAE) score. **Table 1** below shows all RMSE and MAE performances of the implemented models.

The results as displayed in **Table 1** show that five out of six models were able to make better forecasts than the forecasts made by the baseline model. The AR, ES, HWES, ARIMA and CNN model made forecasts that were all slightly or significantly better than the forecast made by the simple average model. Only the moving average (MA) model made forecasts that resulted in almost identical RMSE and MAE error scores, compared to the performances of the baseline model.

The research results show that the 1-D sequential CNN with vector output is the best performing model on the test data. In **Figure 6** the forecasts made by the CNN model are displayed, and clearly show significant alignment with the test data. The models relative good results could indicate that convolutional operations perform well on 1-D sequence data, and are able to make better forecasts than traditional machine learning models. The 1-D sequential CNN made approximately five times more accurate forecasts than the ARIMA model. The CNN model has a RMSE error of 409,86 and a MAE error of 315,99, compared to an RMSE error of 2172,88 and MAE error of 1721,42 from the ARIMA model. The initial set goal of having a CNN model that is able to outperform the prominent and accurate ARIMA model, has been clearly achieved.

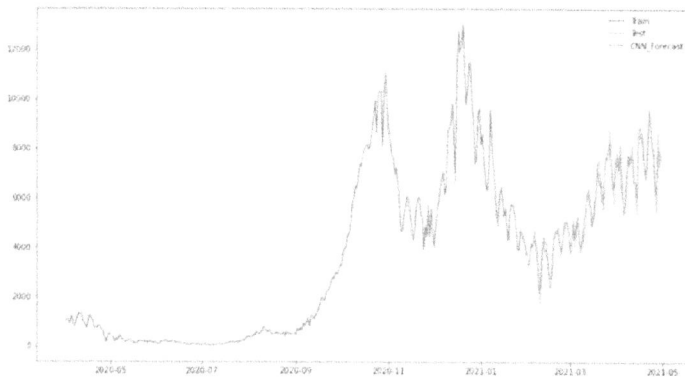

Figure 6.
CNN forecasting performance (green) and actual infections (blue and orange) on the number of corona infections per day, in time interval February – April 2021.

Another favorable model is the Holt-Winters exponential smoothing (HWES) model. With a RMSE error of 1611,34 and MAE error of 1379,34. It performed approximately 25 percent better on the RMSE metric, and made around 20 percent better forecasts according to the MAE metric, than the forecasts made by the ARIMA model. Also the single exponential smoothing (ES) model slightly outperformed the ARIMA model, by about 10 percent.

6. Conclusion

Many sources claim that classical statistical methods, like ARIMA and exponential smoothing, achieve better performance than standard deep learning models, like MLP's and RNN's on smaller datasets.

However, the one-dimensional CNN model with vector output made forecasts that were five time more accurate than the forecasts made by the ARIMA model, on a smaller dataset containing less than one thousand observations. These findings support the fact that neural networks are resistant to errors and some outliers in the underlying dataset, which make them useful in the analysis and prediction of larger and sometimes even smaller time series datasets. Also, classical machine learning methods like ARIMA and exponential smoothing fail to identify and capture nonlinear and complex behavior of time series. Thus, in the case of pandemics, where the data does not show a clear trend and data patterns are relatively hard to extract, neural networks can be a solution for this complexity.

Nevertheless, predicting the future with accurate forecasts is still a very difficult to an even impossible task. This is because of the presence of confounding variables, for example human decision making processes, that cannot be modeled upfront in any of the models. However, the CNN model have proven its potential in predicting and forecasting new corona virus infections. When dealing with viruses that act like COVID-19 in a similar way, artificial neural can, in some cases, simulate future values surprisingly well and close to actual future values.

Abbreviation

ACF	Auto Correlation function
ADF	Augmented Dickey Fuller
AI	artificial intelligence
AIC	Akaike Information Criterion
ANN	artificial neural network
AR	AutoRegressive
ARIMA	AutoRegressive Integrated Moving Average
ARMA	AutoRegressive Moving Average
AutoML	Automatic Machine Learning
CI	computational intelligence
CNN	Convolutional Neural Network
DBN	deep belief network
DRL	deep reinforcement learning
EDA	exploratory data analysis
ES	Exponential smoothing
GRU	Gated Recurrent Unit
HWES	Holt-Winters exponential smoothing
LSTM	Long Short Term Memory
MA	Moving Average

MAE	Mean average error
ML	machine learning
MLP	Multi-Layer Perceptron
PACF	Partial Autocorrelation function
RL	Reinforcement learning
RMSE	Root mean squared error
RNN	Recurrent Neural Network
SGA	Stochastic Gradient Ascent
SGD	Stochastic Gradient Descent

Author details

Steven Kraamwinkel
Vrije Universiteit, Amsterdam, The Netherlands

*Address all correspondence to: stevenkraamwinkel@gmail.com

IntechOpen

References

[1] Papastefanopoulos V, Linardatos P, Kotsiantis S. Covid-19: A Comparison of Time Series Methods to Forecast Percentage of Active Cases per Population. Department of Mathematics, University of Patras, Greece. Multidisciplinary Digital Publishing Institute; 2020. DOI: 10.3390/app10113880

[2] Shastri S, Singh K, Kumar S, Kour P, Mansortra V. Time Series Forecasting of Covid-19 using Deep Learning Models: India-USA Comparitive Case Study. Department of Computer Science & IT, University of Jammu, Jammu & Kashmir, India: Elsevier; 2020. DOI: 10.1016/j.chaos.2020.110227

[3] Goodfellow I, Bengio Y, Courville A. Deep Learning. Cambridge, Massachussetts, USA: MIT Press; 2016. ISBN: 9780262035613. url: http://www.deeplearningbook.org

[4] Brownlee J. Deep Learning for Time Series Forecasting: Predict the Future with MLPs, CNNs and LSTMs in Python. Calle de San Francisco, San Juan, Puerto Rico: Machine Learning Mastery; 2018

[5] Gamboa J. Deep Learning for Time Series Analysis. Germany; University of Kaiserslautern; 2017. arXiv:1701.01887

[6] Hyndman R, Athanasopoulos G. Forecasting: Principles and Practice. OTexts, Melbourne, Australia: Monash University; 2018. ISBN: 978-0-9875071-1-2

[7] NIST/SEMATECH: Engineering statistics handbook. National Institute of Standards and Technology. U.S. Department of Commerce; 2013. DOI: 10.18434/M32189

[8] Yamak P, Yujian L, Gadosey P. A Comparison between Arima, Lstm, and Gru for Time Series Forecasting. In:

Proceedings of 2019 2nd International Conference of Algorithms; 2019. DOI: 10.1145/3377713.3377722

[9] Mather B. Time Series with Python: How to Implement Time Series Analysis and Forecasting Using Python, Massachussetts, USA: Kindle Store, Amazon; 2020. ISBN: 978-0-6487830-7-7

[10] Livieris I, Pintelas E, Pintelas P. A CNN–LSTM Model for Gold Price Time-Series Forecasting. Department of Mathematics, University of Patras, Greece: Springer; 2020. DOI: 10.1007/s00521-020-04867

[11] Pal A, Prakash P. Practical Time Series Analysis: Master Time Series Data Processing, Visualization, and Modeling Using Python. Livery Place, Birmingham, UK: Packt Publishing Ltd,; 2017. ISBN: 978-1-78829-022-7

[12] Döring M. Data science blog. 2020. Available from: https://www.datascienceblog.net/\newlinepost/machine-learning/forecasting_vs_prediction/. [Accessed: April 8, 2021]

[13] Brownlee J: What Is Time Series Forecasting? Machine Learning Mastery Pty Ltd, Calle de San Francisco, San Juan, Puerto Rico; 2016. Available from: https://machinelearningmastery.com/time-series-forecasting. [Accessed: March 17, 2021]

[14] Faloutsos C, Gasthaus J, Januschowski T, Wang Y. Forecasting big Time Series: Old and new. VLDB Endowment. Seattle, Washington, USA: Amazon AI Labs; 2018. DOI: 10.14778/3229863.3229878

[15] Pulagam S: Time Series Forecasting using Auto ARIMA in Python. San Francisco HQ, San Francisco, California, USA: Towards Data Science. Medium Corporation; 2020. Available

from: https://towardsdatascience.com/time-series-forecasting-using-auto\newline-arima-in-python-bb83e49210cd. [Accessed: May 8, 2021]

[16] Shi Q, Yin J, Cichocki A, Yokota T, Chen L, Yuan M, Zeng J. Block Hankel Tensor ARIMA for Multiple Short Time Series Forecasting. New York: 34th AAAI Conference on Artificial Intelligence; 2020. DOI: 10.1609/aaai.v34i04.6032

[17] Petnehazi G. Recurrent Neural Networks for Time Series Forecasting. Doctoral School of Mathematical and Computational Sciences, Hungary: University of Debrecen; 2019. arXiv: 1901.00069v1

[18] Jain A: A Comprehensive Beginner's Guide to Create a Time Series Forecast. Udyog Vihar, Gurugram, India: Analytics Vidhya. 2016. Available from: https://www.analyticsvidhya.com/blog/2016/02/time-series-forecasting-codes-python. [Accessed: April 8, 2021]

[19] Lim B, Zohren S. Time Series Forecasting with deep Learning: A Survey, Oxford, UK: Philosophical Transactions of the Royal Society A; 2020. arXiv:2004.13408; 2020

[20] Kaushik S, Choudhury A, Sheron P, Dasgupta N, Natarajan S, Pickett L, et al. AI in Healthcare: Time-series Forecasting using Statistical, Neural, and Ensemble Architectures, Lausanne, Switzerland: Frontiers in Big Data; 2020. DOI: 10.3389/fdata.2020.00004

[21] Singh A: 7 Methods to Perform Time Series Forecasting. Udyog Vihar, Gurugram, India: Analytics Vidhya; 2018. Available from: https://www.analyticsvidhya.com/blog/2018/02/time-series-forecasting-methods. [Accessed: March 5, 2021]

[22] Hewamalage H, Bergmeir C, Bandara K. Recurrent Neural Networks for time series Forecasting: Current Status and Future Directions. Monash University, Australia: Elsevier; 2021. DOI: 10.1016/j.ijforecast.2020.06.008

[23] Prem: Top 5 common Time Series Forecasting Algorithms. Iunera GmbH & Co KG. 2021. Available from: https://www.iunera.com/kraken/big-data-science-intelligence/time-series-and-analytics/top-5-common-time-series-forecasting\newline-algorithms. [Accessed: May 27, 2021]

[24] Brownlee J: 11 Classical Time Series Forecasting Methods in Python(Cheat Sheet). Calle de San Francisco, San Juan, Puerto Rico: Machine Learning Mastery Pty Ltd; 2018. Available from: https://machinelearningmastery.com/time-series-forecasting-methods-in-\newline python-cheat-sheet. [Accessed: May 8, 2021]

[25] Domingos S, de Oliveira J, de Mattos NF, Paulo S. An Intelligent Hybridization of ARIMA with Machine Learning Models for Time Series Forecasting. Universidade de Pernambuco, Brazil: Elsevier; 2019. DOI: 10.1016/j.knosys.2019.03.011

[26] Masum S, Liu Y, Chiverton J. Multi-step Time Series Forecasting of Electric Load Using Machine Learning Models. University of Portsmouth, UK: Springer; 2018. DOI: 10.1007/978-3-319-91253-0_15

[27] Brownlee J. How to Create an ARIMA Model for Time Series Forecasting in Python. Calle de San Francisco, San Juan, Puerto Rico: Machine Learning Mastery Pty Ltd; 2017. Available from: https://machinelearningmastery.com/arima-for-time-series-forecasting-with_python

[28] McKinney W, Perktold J, Seabold S. Time Series Analysis in Python with Statsmodels. Duke University, Durham, North Carolina, USA: Jarrodmillman Com; 2011

[29] Moews B, Herrmann J, Ibikunle G. Lagged Correlation-Based Deep

Learning for Directional Trend Change Prediction in Financial Time Series. University of Edinburgh, UK: Elsevier; 2019. DOI: 10.1016/j.eswa.2018.11.027

[30] Bishop C. Pattern Recognition and Machine Learning. Cambridge, UK: Springer, Microsoft Research Ltd,; 2006. ISBN-10: 0-387-31073-8

[31] Sezer O, Gudelek M, Ozbayoglu A. Financial Time Series Forecasting with Deep Learning: A Systematic Literature Review: 2005–2019. TOBB University of Economics and Technology, Ankara, Turkey: Elsevier; 2020. DOI: 10.1016/j.asoc.2020.106181

[32] Heller M: Automated Machine Learning or AutoML Explained. Needham, Massachussetts, USA: IDG Communications Inc; 2019. Available from: https://www.infoworld.com/article/3430788/automated-machine-learning-or-\newlineautoml-explained.html. [Accessed: May 27, 2021]

[33] Amidi S. Deep Learning Cheatsheet. Stanford, California, USA: Standford University; 2018. Available from: https://stanford.edu/~shervine/teaching/cs-229/cheatsheet-deep-learning

[34] Bealdung Corporation: Epoch in Neural Networks. Bucharest, Romania; Bealdung; 2021. Available from: https://www.baeldung.com/cs/epoch-neural-networks

[35] LeCun Y, Bengio Y. Convolutional Networks for Images, Speech, and Time Series. The handbook of Brain Theory and Neural Networks. Holmdel, New Jersey, USA: AT&T Bell Laboratories; 1995. Available from: http://www.iro.umontreal.ca/~lisa/pointeurs/handbook-convo.pdf

[36] Pozorska J, Scherer M. Company Bankruptcy Prediction with Neural Networks. Springer, Czestochowa, Poland: Czestochowa University of Technology; 2018. DOI: 10.1007/978-3-319-91253-0_18

[37] Smith J, Wilamowski B. Discrete Cosine Transform Spectral Pooling Layers for Convolutional Neural Networks. Alabama, USA: Springer. Auburn University; 2018. DOI: 10.1007/978-3-319-91253-0_23

[38] Solia P: Convolutions and Backpropagations. San Francisco HQ, San Francisco, California, USA: Medium Corporation; 2018. Available from: https://medium.com/@pavisj/convolutions-and-backpropagations\newline-46026a8f5d2c. [Accessed: May 19, 2021]

[39] Raschka S, Patterson J, Nolet C. Machine Learning in Python: Main Developments and Technology Trends in Data Science, Machine Learning, and Artificial Intelligence. Multidisciplinary Digital Publishing Institute, Madison, Wisconsin, USA: University of Wisconsin-Madison; 2020. DOI: 10.3390/info11040193

[40] Data Science Show: How to use ACF and PACF to Identify Time Series Analysis Models. 2020. Available from: https://www.youtube.com/watch?v=CAT0Y66nPhs&ab_channel=DataScienceShow. [Accessed: May 27, 2021]

[41] Andrade F. A simple Guide to Beautiful Visualizations in Python. San Francisco HQ, San Francisco, California, USA; Medium corporation. Available from: https://towardsdatascience.com/a-simple-guide-to-beautiful-\newlinevisualizations-in-python-\newlinef564e6b9d392. [Accessed: May 8, 2021]

[42] Smyl S. A Hybrid Method of Exponential Smoothing and Recurrent Neural Networks for Time Series Forecasting. San Francisco, California, USA: Elsevier. Uber Technologies; 2020. DOI: 10.1016/j.ijforecast.2019.03.017

[43] Garcia S, Ramirez-Gallego S, Luengo J, Benitez J, Herrera F. Big Data Preprocessing: Methods and Prospects.

BioMed Central, Spain: University of Granada; 2016. DOI: 10.1186/s41044-016-0014-0

[44] Brownlee J: How to Prepare Data for Machine Learning. Calle de San Francisco, San Juan, Puerto Rico: Machine Learning Mastery Pty.; 2020. Available from: https://machinelearningmastery.com/how-to-prepare-data-for-machine\newline-learning/. [Accessed: April 25, 2021]

[45] Watson A: Prediction Vs Forecasting. San Francisco HQ, San Francisco, California, USA: Medium corporation; 2021. Available from: https://towardsdatascience.com/creating-synthetic-time-series-data-\newline67223ff08e34. [Accessed: February 22, 2021]

[46] Influxdata Inc: Time Series Forecasting Methods. San Francisco, California, USA: InfluxData Inc,; 2021. Available from: https://www.influxdata.com/time-series-forecasting-methods. [Accessed: March 17, 2021]

[47] Brownlee J: Time Series Forecasting Performance Measures with Python. Calle de San Francisco, San Juan, Puerto Rico: Machine Learning Mastery Pty Ltd.; 2020. Available from: https://machinelearningmastery.com/time-series-forecasting-performance\newline-measures-with-python/. [Accessed: 2021-03-17]

[48] Ameisen E: Always Start with a Stupid Model, no Exceptions. San Francisco HQ, San Francisco, California, USA: Medium corporation; 2018. Available from: https://blog.insightdatascience.com/always-start-with-a-stupid-model-no\newline-exceptions-3a22314b9aaa. [Accessed: May 8, 2021]

[49] Brownlee J: How to Develop Convolutional Neural Network Models for Time Series Forecasting. Calle de San Francisco, San Juan, Puerto Rico: Machine Learning Mastery Pty Ltd.;

2018. Available from: https://machinelearningmastery.com/how-to-develop-convolutional-neural\newline-network-models-for-time-series\newline-forecasting/. [Accessed: February 28, 2021]

[50] Praveen_1998: What Is a Convolutional Neural Network. Bommanahalli, Bengaluru, India: Intellipaat; 2020. Available from: https://intellipaat.com/community/46826/what-is-kernel-in-cnn. [Accessed: May 11, 2021]

[51] Binkowski M, Gautier M, Donnat P. Autoregressive convolutional neural networks for asynchronous time series. International Conference on Machine Learning. 2018. PMLR;**80**:580-589

[52] Pulagam S: Time Series Forecasting Using Auto ARIMA in Python. San Francisco HQ, San Francisco, California, USA: Medium corporation; 2020. Available from: https://towardsdatascience.com/time-series-forecasting-using-auto\newline-arima-in-python-bb83e49210cd. [Accessed: May 8, 2021]

Chapter 7

Biological Determinants of Emergence of SARS-CoV-2 Variants

Ricardo Izurieta, Tatiana Gardellini, Adriana Campos and Jeegan Parikh

Abstract

In epidemic and pandemic circumstances, mutant RNA viruses go into a Darwinian selection of species with the predominance of the most transmissible, pathogenic, and virulent variants. Nevertheless, our current knowledge about the determinants of emergence of the new mutants is limited. The perspective chapter presents theoretical concepts related to biological determinants responsible for viral mutations or potential variant emergence. A scoping literature review was done in biomedical databases (PubMed, Medline) and google search engine with papers selected based about the book chapter. Public health and governmental agency websites were utilized for most recent information. Molecular determinants, the heterogenic herd immunity achieved by world populations, partial induced natural immunity by the disease, partial artificial immunity caused by incomplete immunization schedules, animal reservoirs, immunosuppression and chemical and biological antiviral therapies can result in genomic mutations combined with immunological selective pressure resulting in emergence of variants of concern. These variants could be resistant to current vaccines and monoclonal antibodies and can influence the future directions of the COVID-19 pandemic. This can be a threat to international health security and thus it is important to increase the genomic surveillance for mutations and research into modified vaccines and monoclonal antibodies against newer antigens to prevent the prolongation of the pandemic.

Keywords: SARS-CoV-2, COVID-19, variants, determinants

1. Introduction

At the time this chapter is being written, the world is still experiencing the Severe Acute Respiratory Syndrome Coronavirus −2 (SARS-CoV-2)/COVID-19 pandemic. The dominant circulating strain of the virus has gone under multiple changes during the pandemic. The initial ancestral strain gave way to the alpha strain which gave way to the delta and omicron strain, which are currently the dominating circulating strains [1]. In addition, there have been emergence of other variants of interests (VOIs) or variants of concern (VOC) such as beta, gamma, P1, P2, lambda, and mu which could be a threat to international health security [1].

The emergence of these variants suggests virus adaptations to various determinants, responsible for the selection of these mutated variants.

This perspective chapter considers different biological determinants capable to contribute to viral mutations and thereby, emergence of new variants and the potential impact of this on the tools (vaccines and antibody therapy) against the SARS-CoV-2. However, it is important to note the determinants mentioned here may not be an exhaustive list of potential mechanisms to induce mutations. This chapter is based on theoretical and fundamental scientific concepts known to be involved from past outbreaks or current case reports from the ongoing pandemic. It is known that biological and environmental, among other determinants may drive viral mutations by different processes or mechanisms. Furthermore, by considering the roles these potential determinants may or already contribute to future SARS-CoV-2 variants we can improve global pandemic responses, saves lives, and contribute to the international health security.

2. Methods

A scoping literature review in search for current topics associated with SARS-CoV-2 or COVID-19 viral replication, adaptations, and biological determinants known to cause variant emergence (e.g., molecular factors, animal reservoirs, immunological factors, etc.) was conducted in biomedical databases such as PubMed, MEDLINE, and Google search engine. Additionally, World Health Organization (WHO), Centers for Disease Control and Prevention (CDC), and Food and Drug Administration (FDA) websites were relied upon to get the most recent information related to content of the chapter. Papers related to the biological determinants commonly associated with viral replication, recombination, adaptation, and immunological seletion were chosen based on the scope of the chapter. Biological determinants of variant emergence and their possible or current implications on the COVID-19 pandemic are presented below.

3. Biological determinants of SARS-CoV-2 variants emergence

3.1 Molecular determinants

3.1.1 Viral replication/recombination

SARS-CoV-2, a beta coronavirus, is a RNA virus using an error-prone RNA-dependent RNA polymerase for replication [2]. The virus encodes a proofreading $3'$ exonuclease (nsp140) but despite this activity, it accumulates genomic changes having a potential to create heterogenous mixture of antigenic proteins resulting in emergence of new variants [2]. The genomic mutation rate of SARS-CoV-2 in humans is estimated at $0.8–2.38 \times 10^{-3}$ nucleotide substitutions per site per year with experimental data suggesting the virus capable of mutating and accumulating changes when it encounters new cell types [3, 4]. Thus, high viral load means high viral replication and thus higher potential for genomic errors due to replication. Along with the replication associated changes, dramatic changes in the virus phenotype can be observed due to genomic recombination in a cell infected with more than one coronavirus [2, 5]. Till now eight recombination events have been observed in SARS-CoV-2 but the frequency of such events is not known [6]. Random errors accumulated during replication/recombination along with population level natural and vaccine induced immunity, play an important role in Darwinian selection of these variants [2].

3.2 Zoonotic determinants

Although the exact precursor of SARS-CoV-2 is unknown, it is established it is of wild origin. The initial December 2019 outbreak in Wuhan, China was linked to the seafood and live animal city market [7]. This market was reported to trade poultry, snakes, hedgehogs, and other wild animals [8].

The different SARS-CoV-2 variants detected in animals including dogs, cats, tigers, lions, minks, and gorillas all had genomes related to the human variant yet had additional mutations. The presence and infection of these animal reservoirs with SARS-CoV-2 virus also increases the possibility of viral mutations/recombinations and emergence of variants. Zoonotic reservoirs capable of carrying and providing an environment for viral multiplication are listed below.

3.2.1 Bats and pangolins

At the beginning of the pandemic bats were declared as the possible SARS-CoV-2 reservoir because of the genomic similarities with other coronaviruses infecting bats [9]. During the initial molecular epidemiological investigations, it was found the SARS-CoV-2 genome had similarities with coronaviruses isolated in *Rhinolophus* bats [10]. In Cambodia, a coronavirus with 93% genomic similarities was detected in horseshoe bats *Rhinolophus shameli*, but this specific bat species does not reside at the location of original SARS-CoV-2 outbreak [11, 12]. Similarly, 200 novel coronaviruses have been identified among bats worldwide [13]. Furthermore, bats are reservoirs for other emerging pathogens like Ebola, Nipah, rabies, Hendra, and rotaviruses [14]. Nevertheless, there are three events contradicting the hypothesis that bats were the initial reservoir from which SARS-CoV-2 jumped into other species: 1) during the beginning of the pandemic bats were hibernating; 2) bats were not sold at the animal market during the initial outbreak; and 3) although other bat coronaviruses have up to 96% genomic similarities, SARS-CoV-2 has not been detected among bat species [15].

The fist isolated variant of SARS-CoV-2 was identified as pangolin-CoV because of similarities with coronaviruses isolated in the carcasses of Malayan pangolins *Manis javanica* [16]. SARS-CoV-2 has 89% nucleotide and 98% amino acid similarities with the pangolin coronavirus genome [17]. Moreover, recent investigations done in other pangolin species conclude the pangolin coronavirus can be the precursor of SARS-CoV-2 because of their high genetic variation and given no coronaviruses were found in pre-COVID-19 pangolin samples [18].

3.2.2 SARS-CoV-2 variants in domestic and wild animals

The virus has been detected in domestic cats and dogs [14]. Therefore, the transmission from humans to domestic animals is plausible. Specifically, the B.1.1.7 (Alpha) variant has been identified in domestic cats as well as in domestic dogs [19]. In contrast it appears that cattle, goats, and sheep are not infected by the virus [20].

Among animals kept in zoos the virus has been detected in gorillas, tigers, pumas, cougars, Asian small-clawed otters, and snow leopards. The genetic variability of SARS-CoV-2 is evident from the 9 genomes identified in tigers, lions, and their keepers [21]. The B.1.1.7 (Alpha) variant has been detected in gorillas, lions, leopards, and tigers [20, 22]. In another study the B.1.617.2 (Delta) variant was reported in Asiatic lions from India [23]. Farmed wild animals have been diagnosed with SARS-CoV-2. Specifically, SARS-CoV-2 has been identified in American minks (*Neovison vison*) and in ferrets (*Musteal furo*) [20].

Therefore, this possibility of emergence of new variants is ever present due to SARS-CoV-2 spread to different ecological environments and newer animal reservoirs resulting in a subsequent risk for spillover into humans and other species.

3.3 Immunological determinants

3.3.1 Herd immunity

Lately, the phrase "Herd Immunity" is constantly brought up in news outlets, in commentaries, opinion pieces, and peer-reviewed articles. First introduced almost 100 years ago, it only recently gained popularity [24]. Although Herd Immunity is now a widely accepted concept, it may take on multiple meanings, each slightly different than the next. Some researchers consider Herd Immunity a threshold of the proportion of immune individuals that leads to a decline in infections or outbreaks [25, 26]. While others may use it to describe the proportion immune to a specific infection among a population or refer to it as a protective immunity pattern [25]. Herd Immunity is most referred to as the reduction of risk, of an infection, to susceptible individuals by the proximity and presence of immune individuals [25]. Herd Immunity may be used interchangeably as "indirect protection" or "herd effect". Regardless of the definition variations, Herd Immunity leads to one outcome – the reduction of infection incidence. This concept, in conjunction with vaccines, has contributed to some of the most important public health achievements in the 20th and 21st century such as the smallpox eradication, polio elimination, and other vaccine-preventable diseases. This section explores the concepts behind Herd Immunity and current and future implications during the COVID-19 pandemic.

3.3.1.1 Theories which constructed herd immunity

Topley and Wilson (1923) were the first to coin the term "Herd Immunity" and specifically look at host resistance in comparison with mass infection. After first mention of Herd Immunity, the term and overall concept started appearing and developing soon after [27–29]. Dudley [27] explored the idea of a "herd" or community and how it could be defined. He defined the idea of "infection pressure" (i.e., fundamental parasite factor) which may be determined by the infectious agent distribution frequency rates which is in the members of the herd [27]. He claimed, infectious pressure reacts with Herd Immunity, the increase of one increases the other and then decreases it to zero. This introduced the idea of needing a minimum amount of Herd Immunity, a threshold, in order to keep the infectious pressure at zero. Furthermore, he mentioned those two factors contributed to the type, quantity, infection speed (i.e., now known as R_0) and the frequency and distribution of cases and their severity [27].

Yet Herd Immunity had one large limitation—to provide protection, a high proportion of the population must be immune to the pathogen. Before immunizations individuals had to survive and pass the pathogen to become immune; depending on the pathogen, likelihood of survival and being left with life-altering morbidities varied. However, as concepts behind Herd Immunity were evolving, vaccinations were becoming a staple of public health practice, allowing a large proportion of the population to be safely immunized against specific pathogens. Vaccination allowed for the fulfillment of Herd Immunity at a much faster rate and safer manner. This allowed for the concepts to be turned into mathematical possibilities.

Before vaccination and Herd Immunity there were two main hypotheses as to why outbreaks would end even though not all susceptible were affected: (1) the agent naturally loses virulence (2) the dynamics between susceptible, infected, and immune [26]. The later hypothesis, prevailed with its mathematical idea of "mass action principle" (MAP) [26]. This principle was based on a simple logical argument in favor of indirect protection given by Herd Immunity and became an epidemiological theoretical cornerstone. Eventually three theories converged into one general theory driving Herd Immunity: MAP, case reproduction rates (later called base reproductive rates [BRR]), and the Reed-Frost heterogenous population simulation approach [26]. The current formula used for Herd Immunity is $H = 1-1/R_0 = (R_0-1)/R_0$, where R_0 is the BRR. H is the Herd Immunity threshold, the proportion of immunes needed in order to reduce incidence and R_0 is derived from the duration of contagiousness of an infected individual, the likelihood of infection per contact between a susceptible person and an infectious person or vector, and the contact rate [30]. The BRR serves as an indicator of the contagiousness of an infectious agent—the higher the R_0, the more transmissible. An $R_0 > 1$ indicates an outbreak will continue, while a $R_0 < 1$ indicates the end of an outbreak, if $R_0 = 1$ then the outbreak is stable [30]. In novel outbreaks, where everyone is susceptible the R_0 defines the infectiousness of a pathogen. However, as individuals pass the infection or become immunized, the number of susceptible decreases and immune increases, and although this does not technically reduce the BRR, because the definition of R_0 assumes a completely susceptible population, one can use the effective reproduction number (R) in lieu, which is similar to R_0 but does not assume complete population susceptibility and, thus, can be estimated with populations with immune members [30]. Efforts aimed at reducing the number of susceptible persons through vaccination would result in a reduction of the R value, rather than R_0 value.

3.3.1.2 Herd immunity in the context of COVID-19

Currently there are multiple vaccines approved internationally for human use and immunization campaigns are urging communities to get vaccinated, therefore reducing the number of susceptible in hopes to achieve herd immunity. However, there are multiple factors to consider in achieving herd immunity from the SARS-CoV-2 virus.

Originally, with an estimated BRR of 2–3, researchers estimated the proportion of the population needed to be immunized to induce Herd Immunity around 50–67% [31–33]. Since then, the emergence of new SARS-CoV-2 variants, most famously the Delta variant, studies suggest a higher BRR (>5) [34, 35] than the alpha variant (2–3) [31–33, 36–39] increasing the vaccination/immune threshold needed in order to achieve a protective effect. An increase in the necessary number of individuals vaccinated propose additional hurdles in reaching Herd Immunity, with the ever-increasing anti-vax movement or individuals acting as "freeloaders" (i.e., individuals who are not vaccinated, yet expect to be protected by the rest of the community being vaccinated).

Secondly, future SARS-CoV-2 variants may mutate enough where the protection offered by the currently available vaccines or natural immunity may no longer suffice. The emergence of the Delta variant showed a reduced vaccine effectiveness compared to the previous variants, which the vaccines were developed from [40, 41]. While currently approved vaccines still provide significant protection from the Delta variant for reduced risk of infection and disease severity, the reduction in vaccine effectiveness is alarming. If emerging variants significantly or completely evade the protection offered by current vaccines or natural immunity, individuals may no longer fall under the immune proportion of the population. An example of this possible situation was reported in Manaus, Brazil, where by December 2020 the population was estimated to have naturally achieved the herd immunity threshold (i.e., before vaccinations were approved and available), estimated at 67%, yet experienced a wave of hospitalizations in January 2021 [42]. This case study further highlighted the limitations with calculating Herd Immunity. Possible reasons for the Manaus outbreak were an overestimation of the immune population, a possible waning immune response, mutants capable of evading responses from previous natural infection, and mutants may have higher transmissibility than previously circulating lineages [42]. Future scenarios where Herd Immunity may not be achievable or severely reduced would be staggering in relation to vaccination campaigns and reaching herd immunity—a grave threat to international health security.

3.3.2 Artificial immunization/natural infection

All COVID-19 vaccines authorized or have received emergency use authorization (EUA) by FDA, EU/EEA, or WHO require a two-dose schedule except for the Janssen vaccines. All these vaccines require a period of 21 days to 12 weeks spacing between the primary and secondary dose [43]. In the early phase of the pandemic to reduce widespread community transmission, logistical issues, and shortages, many countries (e.g., UK, Canada) elected to delay the second dose in the population, thereby increasing the number of individuals with at least one dose. Policies such as the aforementioned in conjunction with waning of immunity after SARS-CoV-2 natural infection may result in large groups of people with only partial immunity against SARS-CoV-2 [43].

The Darwinian selection of variants with mutations for immune escape and its transmission in the community will depend on substantial selection pressure [44]. The greatest potential for the emergence of these immune escape mutations will be in those hosts with highest viral loads (increased mutations) while the greatest selection pressure will be in those with strongest immunological response [2, 44]. The level of immunological protection conferred after first dosage is dependent on the type of vaccine product in addition to the individual characteristics and variant [43]. In individuals with poor immunological response after first dose, there is potential for greater infection burden [44]. These individuals will have higher assumed rates of evolutionary adaptation because of higher viral load and replication. In those individuals with strong but partial immunological response, the infection rates would be lower but evolutionary selection pressure would be large, resulting in high rates of viral adaptations. Previous phylogenic research done on influenza viruses suggested the viral evolution and emergence of immune escape variants is maximum in those individuals with partial immunity (i.e., intermediate levels of selection and viral replication) [45]. Thus, having partially immunized individuals could lead to short-term benefits such as reduced peak of disease but in long term can result in higher infection burden and substantially higher risk of viral evolution to immune escape variants [44].

3.3.2.1 Chemical and biological therapy

Several monoclonal antibodies were developed against the spike protein of SARS-CoV-2 to block the transmission of the virus inside the cells [46]. A single (Bamlanivimab) or combination monoclonal antibodies (Bamlanivimab/Etsevimab or Casirivimab/Imdevimab) received EUA for therapeutic management of SARS-CoV-2 and post-exposure prophylaxis [47, 48]. In theory, administration of monoclonal antibody therapy can alter the immunological selective pressure resulting in viral adaptation for the emergence of variants resistant to one or more monoclonal antibodies [49, 50]. This potential for the emergence of monoclonal antibody resistance has been observed in immunocompromised patients [51–53]. In trials for monoclonal antibodies, mutations resistant to antibodies were detected by next generation sequencing (NGS) assay in 10% of the patients receiving therapy with its transmissibility not determined [54]. Recently, a Wisconsin (WI) study using Bamlanivimab described the emergence of new resistant mutation E484K with further transmission to nearby contacts [55]. The emergence of variants with reduced susceptibility to neutralizing antibodies after polyclonal convalescent plasma therapy provides further proof of the effect of immunological selective pressure on emergence of new variants [49, 56]. It is conceivable, the widespread use of monoclonal or polyclonal antibody therapy may reduce barriers for the emergence of resistant variants to these antibodies which can further transmit to wider communities, potentially becoming a variant of concern. A widespread genomic surveillance is warranted to identify and control the spread of these antibody resistant variants [55].

3.3.3 Immunosuppressed individuals

During evaluation of the efficacy of vaccines, subjects with inhered or acquired immunodeficiencies are excluded from clinical trials. Therefore, there are limited information about the immunogenicity of SARS-CoV-2 vaccines among these patients. Field studies evaluating the effectiveness of COVID-19 vaccines demonstrate that immunocompromised subjects mount a lower antibody response when compared with immunocompetent subjects [57].

Viruses are highly sophisticated molecular machines that can go into an adaptive evolution in the human host establishing a latent reservoir, integrating into the human genome, or causing a chronic infection. Viruses such as hepatitis B virus, hepatitis C virus, and human immunodeficiency virus go into latent stage evading the host immune response while other viruses like Ebola can persist in immune sanctuaries [58]. Considering COVID-19 is an infection of pandemic proportions, it is plausible to think human host immune pressure can contribute to SARS-CoV-2 genetic diversity and selection with phenotypic changes [59]. Consequently, it is necessary to address the relationship between viral persistence in the immunosuppressed host. As a matter of fact, one of the hallmarks of SARS-CoV-2 is its capacity to co-opt various cellular factors and machineries damping the immune response [60]. Although not yet demonstrated, it is plausible to suggest SARS-CoV-2 may establish a latent infection or remain in immune sanctuary. However, SARS-CoV-2 persistence in the immunocompromised patient is well documented [61, 62], with viral persistence reported among cancer patients and transplant recipients [61, 63–67]. Viral coronavirus RNA has been detected up to ~60 days in cancer patients that developed respiratory symptoms. Moreover, the longest persistence of coronavirus RNA is recorded at 151 days in a patient with anti-phospholipid syndrome, which suggest these pathogens are of the opportunistic characteristic [68–70]. In the aforementioned patient, there were 31 substitutions and 3 deletions identified in the genome sequences from the isolated agent. There were 12 mutations in the spike protein including 7 in the receptor-binding domain segment. Due to severe pulmonary complication the patient died [71]. Increased viral changes were also detected in another immunocompromised patient, whose disease prolonged for 101 days, where viral changes were limited during the first 60 days but increased after receiving plasma form a convalescent patient at days 63 and 65. Moreover, rapid shifts were observed in the spike area during the last days of the monitoring [71]. In another case-series, three patients receiving chimeric antigen receptor (CAR) T cells because of B-cell acute lymphocytic leukemia, showed multiple escape SARS-CoV-2 variants [71]. Consequently, like SARS-CoV-2 longer persistence in immunosuppressed patients, immunosusceptible elderly patients may also harbor the virus for prolonged periods compared to immunocompetent patients. Gaspar-Rodriguez et al. enunciated in 2021 that SARS-CoV-2 and other coronaviruses potentially establish a long-term, non-productive persistent infection in epithelial, myeloid, and neural host cells until viral clearance is achieved [62]. Prolonged COVID-19 in the immunosuppressed patient can be a determinant of the development of SARS-CoV-2 variants which can be spread among the general population [71]. This persistence of the virus in different types of immunosuppression are listed below.

3.3.3.1 SARS-CoV-2 in Cancer patients

Cancer patients are in immunodepression conditions because of the malignancy and oncological treatments like chemotherapy, radiotherapy, transplants, and immunotherapy. Patients with lung, blood, and bone marrow carcinomas are at a higher risk of harboring the virus for prolonged periods when compared with other cancer patients [72]. Patients with chronic lymphocytic leukemia (CLL) have shown inadequate levels of antibodies as well as cellular immune response [73]. These inadequate immune responses in CLL patients correlates with severe and prolonged forms of COVID-19 and has been supported by late conversion to negative PCR monitoring tests and longer hospitalizations [74]. The impaired humoral and cellular immune response in the CLL patients make these patients long term shedders of SARS-CoV-2 until infection is passed. One case study showed a COVID-19 positive CLL patient having persistent positive PCR test for 105 days after diagnosis [63]. Moreover, during this period a continuous variability in predominant viral variants was observed [63]. This delay in viral clearance in COVID-19 patients has been observed in patients receiving intravenous immunoglobulins as well as in those with hypertension [75].

3.3.3.2 SARS-CoV-2 in organ transplant patients

Organ transplant recipients are patients with long-lasting immunosuppression; therefore, organ transplant recipients have been declared subjects with high risk for severe COVID-19. When COVID-19 positive liver transplant patients were compared with COVID-19 immunocompetent patients, the transplant recipients showed lower prevalence of antibodies against SARS-CoV-2, as well as a faster antibody decline [57]. Regarding viral shedding, immunocompetent asymptomatic COVID-19 infection subjects experience a faster viral clearance when compared with symptomatic individuals [76]. Kidney transplant patients with immunosuppression showed a longer shedding of the virus, of more than 28 days, which was correlated with a prolongation of symptoms [77].

3.3.3.3 SARS-CoV-2 in elderly patients

It is demonstrated SARS-CoV-2 causes highest mortality among elderly populations. Also, viral shedding is increased, enhancing the spread of the virus as it was observed in the increased transmission in nursing homes. An explanation for these complications may be due to the elderly immune system being less competent than in young populations. In the elderly, it appears the production of cytokine and T-cells production worsen the inflammation process especially among those with comorbidities [78]. The increased shedding of SARS-CoV-2 is associated with a more severe clinical presentation and higher viral load peaks [79–81]. The delayed viral clearance in elderly patients' airways can be explained by a decreased respiratory muscle function and diminished mucociliary function [79, 82].

3.3.3.4 SARS-CoV-2 in patients with corticosteroid treatment

Although corticosteroid therapy is being used to ameliorate the inflammation process, the use of corticosteroids at an early stage can suppress the immune cells which can prolong the clearance of the virus as well as its shedding. In a randomized study in the patients without respiratory failure, the methylprednisolone group showed a median viral shedding of 10 days vs. 6 days in the control group [83].

4. Discussion

The molecular mechanisms of viral replication, multiple animal reservoirs, and immunological selection methods have the possibility for viral evolution to immune escape variants (**Figure 1**). Such epidemiological and evolutionary mechanisms are already seen in the emergence of different VOC worldwide [44].

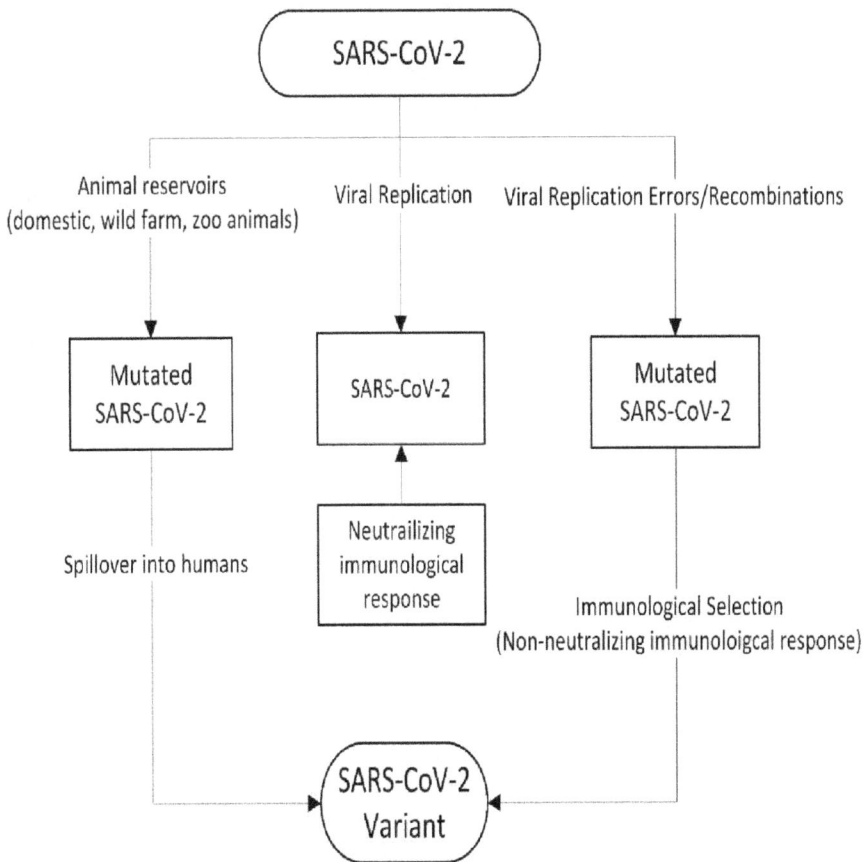

Figure 1.
Biological determinants of emergence of SARS-CoV-2 variants. An infection of SARS-CoV-2 in humans results in viral replication. In born errors of viral replication or genomic recombination can result in viral mutations. People with natural/artificial immunity will neutralize the non-mutated virus but has non-neutralizing immune response against mutated variant. Mutated SARS-CoV-2 thus undergoes this immunological selection for emergence of SARS-CoV-2 variant. Infection in animals with different host cell machinery led to mutated SARS-CoV-2 with potential for species jump and spillover into humans and emergence of SARS-CoV-2 variant.

4.1 Impact of emergence of new variants on vaccine

Since the beginning of the pandemic, VOC having selective advantage of more transmissibility and resistance to natural or vaccine induced immunity have been evolving and supplanting previously circulating strains [43, 84]. The emergence of these VOC affects the effectiveness of vaccines in both partially and fully immunized individuals [43]. In vitro studies demonstrated lower neutralization capacity against all VOC compared to ancestral strains [41, 85, 86]. Based on evidence available for all vaccine types, partially immunized individuals have a lower degree of protection against symptomatic infection, moderate disease, and probable transmission with Delta VOC than Alpha VOC. In general, the vaccine effectiveness for all variants against symptomatic disease was much lower than those reported against severe diseases. The fully immunized individuals confer nearly equivalent protection for all outcomes against Alpha to that of Delta variants [43]. **Table 1** summarizes the results of vaccine effectiveness by type of vaccine, outcome, and VOC.

The emergence of new vaccine-resistant variants may necessitate the development of modified vaccines based on new sequences to prevent the prolonged circulation of vaccine-resistant variants [84]. It is important to conduct studies of these modified vaccines to determine its efficacy in developing a neutralizing immunological response against vaccine-resistant variants. This research is important despite the deployment of these newer vaccines not required until there is evidence of failure of current vaccines. Once the modified vaccines are introduced the molecular and immunological determinants of viral adaptation will necessitate to repeat the cycle of monitoring for even newer variants that might require further modifications in the antigenic sequence in vaccines.

4.2 Impact of emergence of new variants antibody therapy

Like vaccines, the viral adaptations seen against the monoclonal antibody therapy can complicate the deployment of these treatments at large scale in the general

Variant	Original	Original	Alpha	Beta	Gamma	Delta	Delta
Vaccine	SI	SD	SI	SI	SI	SI	SD
Comirnaty (Pfizer/ BioNTech)	95%	100%	89.5%	75%	61%	87.9%	96%
SpikeVax (Moderna)	94.1%	100%	↓ Ant Neu	↓ Ant Neu	↓ Ant Neu	↓ Ant Neu	
Vaxzeria (AstraZeneca)	70.4%	81.3%	66.1%	10.4%	↓ Ant Neu	59.8%	92%
Johnson & Johnson	74.2%	85.4%		64%	↓ Ant Neu		
Cansino		90–95%					
Sputnik V	91.6%	100%	No difference	↓ Ant Neu			
Sinovac	78.1%	100%	↓ Ant Neu	↓ Ant Neu	↓ Ant Neu		
Soberana (Cuba)	62%						

SI, symptomatic disease; SD, Severe disease.

Table 1.
Vaccine effectiveness of two dose of vaccines against symptomatic infection and severe disease caused by non-VOCs, alpha, and Delta VOCs.

population [55]. The initial widespread use of Bamlanivimab as a single therapy and later removal due to epidemiologic trend further provides evidence for judicious use of monoclonal antibody therapy [87]. The usage of cocktail of antibodies should in theory reduce the probability of random selection of resistant variants however it does not totally remove this possibility [55]. This combined with monoclonal antibodies not preventing transmission, not providing immediate cure, lacking durable immunity, and potentially leading to antibody strains with some cross-resistance against vaccine or natural-acquired immunity suggests the need for caution before widespread usage of monoclonal antibody therapy [41, 55]. Increasing the scale of surveillance for mutations along with research into monoclonal antibodies against newer antigens should be adopted if the scale of use of monoclonal antibody has to be expanded [55].

Thus, the determinants of emergence of SARS-CoV-2 variants necessitates the inclusion of epidemiological, evolutionary, clinical, animal, and in vitro data related to changing antigenic sequences, vaccine and monoclonal antibody efficacy in the decision making of which antigens to be included in vaccines or targeted for therapy [84]. Lastly, it is important to recognize the limitations of the concepts presented in this chapter. This is a prospective chapter piece using concepts and theoretical ideologies commonly attributed to variant emergence. The inclusion of the determinants presented are a combination of expert knowledge on behalf of the authors and a scoping literature review conducted on SARS-CoV-2 and its current variants, therefore, this chapter is not meant to replace a systematic review.

5. Conclusion

This chapter presents theoretical and current determinants for variant emergence, specifically for SAR-CoV-2. The emergence of different VOC through the evolutionary cycle of the SARS-CoV-2 virus during the current pandemic (2019-ongoing) makes it important to understand the biological determinants of new emerging variants. The inherent errors in viral replication in humans and animal reservoirs combined with immunological selective pressure result in the Darwinian selection of variants of SARS-CoV-2 with potential for higher transmissibility and resistance to vaccine-based immunity or monoclonal antibodies. The different types of vaccines and associated immune response, partial immunization, waning of immunity, and heterogenicity in worldwide immunity results in wide differences in immunological selective pressure based on regions and virus evolutions. The global inequality in vaccine distribution further complicates this immunological selection pressure. The epidemiological and evolutionary cycle can result in viral adaptations with potential for selection of variants with higher transmissibility and immune escape properties. The emergence of these dangerous new variants can influence vaccine and antibody therapy effectiveness necessitating modifications in antigenic sequences used in production. This emergence of novel variants thus is a concern for international health security with a potential for furthering the COVID-19 pandemic and its associated negative health, economic, and social effects.

Author details

Ricardo Izurieta*, Tatiana Gardellini, Adriana Campos and Jeegan Parikh
College of Public Health, University of South Florida, Tampa, Florida, United States

*Address all correspondence to: ricardoi@usf.edu

IntechOpen

References

[1] World Health Organization. Tracking SARS-CoV-2 variants. 2021. Available from: https://www.who.int/en/activities/tracking-SARS-CoV-2-variants/ [Accessed 31-10-2021]

[2] Banerjee A, Mossman K, Grandvaux N. Molecular determinants of SARS-CoV-2 variants. Trends in Microbiology. 2021;**29**(10):871-873

[3] Massimo A.et al. Mutation rate of SARS-CoV-2 and emergence of mutators during experimental evolution, Evolution, Medicine, and Public Health. 2022;**10**(1):142-155

[4] De Maio N et al. Mutation rates and selection on synonymous mutations in SARS-CoV-2. Genome Biology and Evolution. 2021;**13**(5):1-14

[5] Lai MM et al. Recombination between nonsegmented RNA genomes of murine coronaviruses. Journal of Virology. 1985;**56**(2):449-456

[6] Pollett S et al. A comparative recombination analysis of human coronaviruses and implications for the SARS-CoV-2 pandemic. Scientific Reports. 2021;**11**(1):17365

[7] Islam A, et al. Transmission dynamics and susceptibility patterns of SARS-CoV-2 in domestic, farmed and wild animals: Sustainable One Health surveillance for conservation and public health to prevent future epidemics and pandemics. Transboundary and Emerging Diseases. 2021 Oct:1-21. https://doi.org/10.1111/tbed.14356

[8] Montagutelli X et al. The B1.351 and P.1 variants extend SARS-CoV-2 host ange to mice. bioRxiv. 2021:1-16. https://doi.org/10.1101/2021.03.18.436013

[9] Ashour HM et al. Insights into the recent 2019 novel coronavirus (SARS-CoV-2) in light of past human coronavirus outbreaks. Pathogens. 2020;**9**(3):186

[10] Wong G et al. Zoonotic origins of human coronavirus 2019 (HCoV-19 / SARS-CoV-2): Why is this work important? Zoological Research. 2020;**41**(3):213-219

[11] Delaune D et al. A novel SARS-CoV-2 related coronavirus in bats from Cambodia. Nature Communications. 2021 Nov 9;**12**(1):6563

[12] Lin XD et al. Extensive diversity of coronaviruses in bats from China. Virology. 2017;**507**:1-10

[13] Chen L et al. DBatVir: The database of bat-associated viruses. Database. 2014;**2014**:bau021

[14] Islam A et al. Epidemiology and molecular characterization of rotavirus a in fruit bats in Bangladesh. EcoHealth. 2020;**17**(3):398-405

[15] Jo WK et al. Potential zoonotic sources of SARS-CoV-2 infections. Transboundary and Emerging Diseases. 2021;**68**(4):1824-1834

[16] Liu P et al. Are pangolins the intermediate host of the 2019 novel coronavirus (SARS-CoV-2)? PLoS Pathogens. 2020;**16**(5):e1008421

[17] Zhang C et al. Protein structure and sequence reanalysis of 2019-nCoV genome refutes snakes as its intermediate host and the unique similarity between its spike protein insertions and HIV-1. Journal of Proteome Research. 2020;**19**(4):1351-1360

[18] Lee J et al. No evidence of coronaviruses or other potentially zoonotic viruses in Sunda pangolins (Manis javanica) entering the wildlife trade via Malaysia. EcoHealth. 2020;**17**(3):406-418

[19] Hamer SA et al. SARS-CoV-2 B.1.1.7 variant of concern detected in a pet dog and cat after exposure to a person with COVID-19, USA. Transboundary and Emerging Diseases. 2022 May;**69**(3):1656-1658

[20] World Organization for Animal Health, Special Survival Commission, and W.H.S. Group, Guidelines for Working with Free-Ranging Wild Mammals in the era of the COVID-19 Pandemic. 2020

[21] McAloose D et al. From people to Panthera: Natural SARS-CoV-2 infection in tigers and lions at the Bronx zoo. MBio. 2020;**11**(5):1-13

[22] Service, A.a.P.H.I. Confirmation of COVID-19 in Otters at an Aquarium in Georgia. U.S. U.S. Department of Agriculture; 2021

[23] Mishra A et al. SARS-CoV-2 Delta Variant among Asiatic Lions, India. Emerging Infectious Diseases. 2021;**27**(10):2723-2725

[24] Topley WW, Wilson GS. The spread of bacterial infection. The problem of herd-immunity. The Journal of Hygiene. 1923;**21**(3):243-249

[25] Fine P, Eames K, Heymann DL. "herd immunity": A rough guide. Clinical Infectious Diseases. 2011;**52**(7):911-916

[26] Fine PE. Herd immunity: History, theory, practice. Epidemiologic Reviews. 1993;**15**(2):265-302

[27] Dudley SF. Human adaptation to the parasitic environment. Proceedings of the Royal Society of Medicine. 1929;**22**(5):569-592

[28] Halliday JL. The epidemiology of poliomyelitis. Glasgow Medical Journal. 1931;**115**(3):121-134

[29] Stocks P. Infectiousness and immunity in regard to chickenpox, whooping-cough,

diphtheria, scarlet fever and measles. Proceedings of the Royal Society of Medicine. 1930;**23**(9):1349-1368

[30] Delamater PL et al. Complexity of the basic reproduction number (R(0)). Emerging Infectious Diseases. 2019;**25**(1):1-4

[31] Kwok KO et al. Herd immunity - estimating the level required to halt the COVID-19 epidemics in affected countries. Journal of Infection. 2020;**80**(6):e32-e33

[32] Randolph HE, Barreiro LB. Herd immunity: Understanding COVID-19. Immunity. 2020;**52**(5):737-741

[33] Syal K. COVID-19: Herd immunity and convalescent plasma transfer therapy. Journal of Medical Virology. 2020;**92**(9):1380-1382

[34] Dyer O. Covid-19: Delta infections threaten herd immunity vaccine strategy. BMJ. 2021;**374**:n1933

[35] Liu Y, Rocklöv J. The reproductive number of the Delta variant of SARS-CoV-2 is far higher compared to the ancestral SARS-CoV-2 virus. Journal of Travel Medicine. 2021;**28**(7):1-3

[36] Billah MA, Miah MM, Khan MN. Reproductive number of coronavirus: A systematic review and meta-analysis based on global level evidence. PLoS One. 2020;**15**(11):e0242128

[37] Chen J et al. Herd immunity and COVID-19. European Review for Medical and Pharmacological Sciences. 2020;**24**(8):4064-4065

[38] Griffin S. Covid-19: Herd immunity is "unethical and unachievable," say experts after report of 5% seroprevalence in Spain. BMJ. 2020;**370**:m2728

[39] Jung F et al. Herd immunity or suppression strategy to combat

COVID-19. Clinical Hemorheology and Microcirculation. 2020;**75**(1):13-17

[40] Lopez Bernal J et al. Effectiveness of Covid-19 vaccines against the B.1.617.2 (Delta) variant. New England Journal of Medicine. 2021;**385**(7):585-594

[41] Planas D et al. Reduced sensitivity of SARS-CoV-2 variant Delta to antibody neutralization. Nature. 2021;**596**(7871):276-280

[42] Sabino EC et al. Resurgence of COVID-19 in Manaus, Brazil, despite high seroprevalence. Lancet. 2021;**397**(10273):452-455

[43] European Center for Disease Control and Prevention. Partial COVID-19 Vaccination, Vaccination Following SARS-CoV-2 Infection and Heterologous Vaccination Schedule: Summary of Evidence. ECDC: Stockholm; 2021

[44] Saad-Roy CM et al. Epidemiological and evolutionary considerations of SARS-CoV-2 vaccine dosing regimes. Science. 2021;**372**(6540):363-370

[45] Grenfell BT et al. Unifying the epidemiological and evolutionary dynamics of pathogens. Science. 2004;**303**(5656):327-332

[46] Lloyd EC, Gandhi TN, Petty LA. Monoclonal antibodies for COVID-19. JAMA. 2021;**325**(10):1015-1015

[47] U.S. Food and Drug Adminsitration. FDA Authorizes Monoclonal Antibodies for Treatment of COVID-19. 2020

[48] U.S. Food and Drug Adminsitration, FDA authorizes bamlanivimab and etesevimab monoclonal antibody therapy for post-exposure prophylaxis (prevention) for COVID-19. 2021

[49] Colson P et al. A possible role of Remdesivir and plasma therapy in the selective sweep and emergence of new

SARS-CoV-2 variants. Journal of Clinical Medicine. 2021;**10**(15):3276

[50] Kreuzberger N et al. SARS-CoV-2-neutralising monoclonal antibodies for treatment of COVID-19. Cochrane Database of Systematic Reviews. 2021;**9**(9):Cd013825

[51] Jensen B et al. Emergence of the E484K mutation in SARS-COV-2-infected immunocompromised patients treated with bamlanivimab in Germany. The Lancet Regional Health–Europe. 2021;**8**:100164

[52] Lohr B et al. Bamlanivimab Treatment Leads to Rapid Selection of Immune Escape Variant Carrying the E484K Mutation in a B.1.1.7-Infected and Immunosuppressed Patient. Clinical Infectious Diseases. 6 Dec 2021;**73**(11):2144-2145

[53] Peiffer-Smadja N et al. Emergence of E484K mutation following Bamlanivimab monotherapy among High-risk patients infected with the alpha variant of SARS-CoV-2. Viruses.2021;**13**(8):1642

[54] Chen P et al. SARS-CoV-2 neutralizing antibody LY-CoV555 in outpatients with Covid-19. New England Journal of Medicine. 2020;**384**(3):229-237

[55] Sabin AP et al. Acquisition and onward transmission of a SARS-CoV-2 E484K variant among household contacts of a bamlanivimab- treated patient. medRxiv. 2021: 1-14. https://doi.org/10.1101/2021.10.02.21264415

[56] Andreano E et al. SARS-CoV-2 escape from a highly neutralizing COVID-19 convalescent plasma. Proceedings of the National Academy of Sciences. 2021;**118**(36):e2103154118

[57] Deborska-Materkowska D, Kaminska D. The immunology of SARS-CoV-2 infection and vaccines in

solid organ transplant recipients. Viruses. 2021;**13**(9):1879

[58] Zhou Y et al. Viral (hepatitis C virus, hepatitis B virus, HIV) persistence and immune homeostasis. Immunology. 2014;**143**(3):319-330

[59] Centers for Disease Control and Prevention. Science Brief: Emerging SARS-CoV-2 Variants. 2021. Available from: https://www.cdc.gov/ coronavirus/2019-ncov/science/ science-briefs/scientific-brief-emerging-variants.html [Accessed 30-10-2021]

[60] Desimmie BA et al. Insights into SARS-CoV-2 persistence and its relevance. Viruses. 2021;**13**(6):1025

[61] Fung M, Babik JM. COVID-19 in immunocompromised hosts: What we know so far. Clinical Infectious Diseases. 2021;**72**(2):340-350

[62] Gaspar-Rodriguez A, Padilla-Gonzalez A, Rivera-Toledo E. Coronavirus persistence in human respiratory tract and cell culture: An overview. The Brazilian Journal of Infectious Diseases. 2021;**25**(5):101632

[63] Avanzato VA et al. Case study: Prolonged infectious SARS-CoV-2 shedding from an asymptomatic immunocompromised individual with Cancer. Cell. 2020;**183**(7):1901-1912 e9

[64] Decker A et al. Prolonged SARS-CoV-2 shedding and mild course of COVID-19 in a patient after recent heart transplantation. American Journal of Transplantation. 2020;**20**(11): 3239-3245

[65] Moore JL et al. A 63-year-old woman with a history of non-Hodgkin lymphoma with persistent SARS-CoV-2 infection who was seronegative and treated with convalescent plasma. American Journal of Case Reports. 2020;**21**:e927812

[66] Nakajima Y et al. Prolonged viral shedding of SARS-CoV-2 in an immunocompromised patient. Journal of Infection and Chemotherapy. 2021;**27**(2):387-389

[67] Wei L et al. Prolonged shedding of SARS-CoV-2 in an elderly liver transplant patient infected by COVID-19: A case report. Annals of Palliative Medicine. 2021;**10**(6):7003-7007

[68] Choi B et al. Persistence and evolution of SARS-CoV-2 in an immunocompromised host. New England Journal of Medicine. 2020;**383**(23):2291-2293

[69] Dominguez SR, Robinson CC, Holmes KV. Detection of four human coronaviruses in respiratory infections in children: A one-year study in Colorado. Journal of Medical Virology. 2009;**81**(9):1597-1604

[70] Ogimi C et al. Prolonged shedding of human coronavirus in hematopoietic cell transplant recipients: Risk factors and viral genome evolution. The Journal of Infectious Diseases. 2017;**216**(2): 203-209

[71] Corey L et al. SARS-CoV-2 variants in patients with immunosuppression. New England Journal of Medicine. 2021;**385**(6):562-566

[72] Pratapa SK et al. Caring for Cancer patients during Corona pandemic-(COVID-19)-a narrative review. South Asian Journal of Cancer. 2021;**10**(1): 19-22

[73] Mihaila RG. Management of patients with chronic lymphocytic leukemia during the SARS-CoV-2 pandemic. Oncology Letters. 2021;**22**(2):636

[74] Paneesha S et al. Covid-19 infection in therapy-naive patients with B-cell chronic lymphocytic leukemia. Leukemia Research. 2020;**93**:106366

[75] Chen X et al. Risk factors for the delayed viral clearance in COVID-19

patients. Journal of Clinical Hypertension (Greenwich, Conn.). 2021;**23**(8):1483-1489

[76] Cevik M et al. SARS-CoV-2, SARS-CoV, and MERS-CoV viral load dynamics, duration of viral shedding, and infectiousness: A systematic review and meta-analysis. The Lancet Microbe. 2021;**2**(1):e13-e22

[77] Laracy JC, Miko BA, Pereira MR. The solid organ transplant recipient with SARS-CoV-2 infection. Current Opinion in Organ Transplantation. 2021;**26**(4):412-418

[78] Smorenberg A et al. How does SARS-CoV-2 targets the elderly patients? A review on potential mechanisms increasing disease severity. European Journal of Internal Medicine. 2021;**83**:1-5

[79] Ho JC et al. The effect of aging on nasal Mucociliary clearance, beat frequency, and ultrastructure of respiratory cilia. American Journal of Respiratory and Critical Care Medicine. 2001;**163**(4):983-988

[80] Liu Y et al. Viral dynamics in mild and severe cases of COVID-19. The Lancet Infectious Diseases. 2020;**20**(6):656-657

[81] To KK-W et al. Temporal profiles of viral load in posterior oropharyngeal saliva samples and serum antibody responses during infection by SARS-CoV-2: An observational cohort study. The Lancet Infectious Diseases. 2020;**20**(5):565-574

[82] Svartengren M, Falk R, Philipson K. Long-term clearance from small airways decreases with age. The European Respiratory Journal. 2005;**26**(4):609-615

[83] Tang X et al. Early use of corticosteroid may prolong SARS-CoV-2 shedding in non-intensive care unit patients with COVID-19 pneumonia:

A Multicenter, single-blind, randomized control trial. Respiration. 2021;**100**(2):116-126

[84] Krause PR et al. SARS-CoV-2 variants and vaccines. New England Journal of Medicine. 2021;**385**(2):179-186

[85] Liu C et al. Reduced neutralization of SARS-CoV-2 B.1.617 by vaccine and convalescent serum. Cell. 2021;**184**(16):4220-4236.e13

[86] Yadav PD et al. Neutralization of Beta and Delta variant with sera of COVID-19 recovered cases and vaccinees of inactivated COVID-19 vaccine BBV152/Covaxin. Journal of Travel Medicine. 2021;**28**(7):1-3

[87] U.S. Food and Drug Administration, FDA Revokes Emergency Use Authorization for Monoclonal Antibody Bamlanivimab. U.S. FDA: Silver Spring, MD,U.S.; 2021

Section 3

Miscellaneous Topics

Chapter 8

Resilient Health System and Hospital Disaster Planning

Stephen C. Morris

Abstract

Disaster planning is integral component of hospital operations and management, and hospital resiliency is critical to society and health systems following a disaster. Additionally, hospitals, like all public institutions have significant risk of security incidents including terrorism, isolated and mass violence, social unrest, theft and vandalism, natural and human made disasters. Security and disaster planning are cumbersome, expensive and easy to deprioritize. When a hospital disaster is defined as anything that exceeds the limits of the facility to function at baseline, disasters and security incidents are intertwined: disasters create security problems and vice-versa. Hospital resiliency to disasters and security incidents stems from a systems-based approach, departmental and administrative participation, financial investment and flexibility. Significant best practices and lessons learned exist regarding disaster and security planning and ignorance or lack of adoption is tantamount to dereliction of duty on the part of responsible entities. This chapter consists of a review of the concepts of hospital disaster and security planning, response and recovery, as well as hospital specific disaster and security threats (risk) and their associated mitigations strategies. Risks will be presented follow a hazard vulnerability analysis (HVA), a common framework in emergency management, disaster planning and disaster medicine. As such, each element of risk is defined in terms of likelihood and impact of an event. Concepts of disaster medicine that are also addressed, as are administrative concerns, these elements are designed to be applicable to non-experts with an emphasis on cross disciplinary understanding. Additionally, elements are presented using incident and hospital incident command terminology and those not familiar should learn these concepts though free online training on the incident command system provided by several sources including The United States Federal Emergency Management Agency (FEMA), prior to reading.

Keywords: hospital security, disaster management, disaster medicine, disaster preparedness

1. Introduction

Disaster defined. A serious disruption of the functioning of a community or a society at any scale due to hazardous events interacting with conditions of exposure, vulnerability and capacity, leading to one or more of the following: human, material, economic and environmental losses and impacts. -United Nations international strategy for disaster reduction (UNISDR).

Security events involving healthcare are timeless. Examples of security threats include families seeking retribution for perceived substandard care and healthcare facilities seen as military targets during times of conflict, despite universal agreement on medical neutrality [1]. Terrorism and acts of violence against healthcare workers and healthcare institutions are common enough to have become a field of study. There is also some evidence that the trend is growing, and there are many efforts, globally and locally to address the problem [2]. With violence all to common, it is no coincidence that government, policy and security institutions focus much attention on healthcare.

Disasters, from natural and human created events, are defined by the disruption of normal functioning. When the disaster affects multiple social institutions, healthcare's role in society often expands. In such events, for example, hospitals function beyond the provision of healthcare: a refuge for those in need, a gateway to social services, a bellwether for societal wellbeing, a bastion of hope and communal security in the face of disruption. As such the effect of disasters and security incidents on hospitals has an additive physical and psychological effect on the population. From a practical standpoint, the populations access to health services are interrupted or they may choose to avoid care. Additionally, they may have an inherent sense of insecurity as a major and essential public entity has been attacked or disturbed. The resiliency of hospitals, in the face of major disaster and security events, is paramount to social functioning at many levels and as such is a major concern for public officials and citizens through society.

Hospital security has many elements consistent with security of other institutions and organizations as well as many unique areas of vulnerability. Common security elements include basic building security, employment security, asset and material security, crowd and social unrest security, basic disaster specific security and basic IT security. These elements are addressed largely commiserate with standard practices for public institutions and will not be addressed here. Unique security vulnerabilities of hospitals are too many to name and addressing them all is beyond the scope of this text. Additionally, very specific hospital vulnerabilities such as medical waste, unaccompanied minors, and radiation security among others will not be addressed. Major unique vulnerabilities of hospitals largely stem from their reliance on other public institutions, such as governance and businesses, and the central role they play in society.

2. Emergency management, the disaster cycle and a healthcare perspective on security

2.1 Emergency management and disaster medicine

Disaster medicine and emergency management are two separate fields with overlapping areas of influence, like Venn diagrams with a large portion of common space. Therefore, it is critical that one understand the basic principles of emergency management as it relates to healthcare and hospital preparedness and response. The field of emergency management is premised on several paradigms: disasters are predictable, the disaster cycle, command and control and an all hazards approach.

2.2 Disasters are predictable

The idea of disasters being predictable is confounding to the lay public. Taking time to understand that most disasters are predicable with regards to their occurrence, impact and recovery is paramount to appropriate planning, response and recovery. Furthermore, identifying what element of disaster are not predictable also allows for appropriate planning and should be acknowledged.

Examples of disaster Predictability	Examples of disaster elements that are unpredictable:
Hurricanes will affect the Caribbean between July and October	Timing of events.
Structurally unsound buildings will be damaged in an earthquake	Terrorist activities.
Social unrest will increase healthcare usage and burden of disease.	Storm trajectory, intensity and impact
Post disaster communal living conditions result in increased risk of communicable disease.	Earthquake timing, intensity and effect.

2.3 The disaster cycle

Together with the disasters themselves, institutions and societal response to disasters is predicable. This predictability has two patterns: the disaster cycle, and the social perception of disasters.

The disaster cycle refers to a pattern of institutional behavior surrounding disasters [3]. Since this is a cycle, one must appreciate the continuum and the interconnectedness of the elements. While the terms used change, the basic concepts of event, movement back to normal function, analysis of the event, mitigation, and preparedness remain the same through the fields of disaster medicine and disaster management.

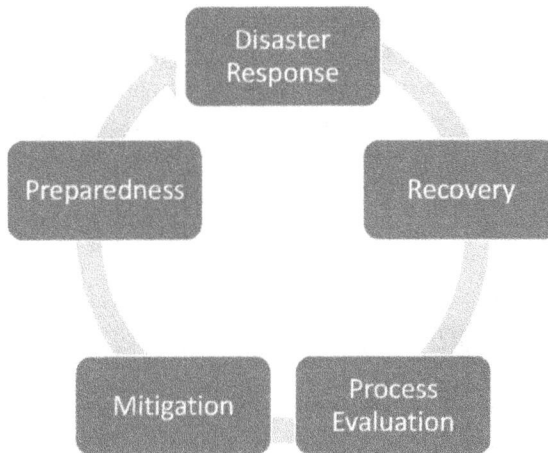

2.3.1 Disaster response

The most publicly visible part of the cycle, the response phase, attempts to control the chaos of the acute period immediately following a disaster event. An event that overwhelms the health system, the definition of a disaster, necessitates adaption of the health system. From a hospital and health systems standpoint, this usually entails attempts to maintain the standard of care, provide for disaster victims and chronic illnesses, and support the greater community. The response period is undefined- from hours in the case of a mass casualty incident to years in the setting of armed conflict or humanitarian crisis.

2.3.2 Recovery

This phase of the disaster cycle is the period taken from the end of the disaster response phase, as defined by stabilizing of the situation, to the return of normal function. From a health systems standpoint, restoration of all services, provision of normal care including elective care, financial and administrative normalization are all goals of the recover period.

2.3.3 Process evaluation

Often left out of the disaster cycle is the appreciation of the interpretation of actions during the disaster response and recovery periods. It is from this analysis, that the lessons learned from the response and recovery are adapted into the foundations of mitigation and preparedness. Without establishing an understanding of systemic successes and failure, mistakes will be repeated.

2.3.4 Mitigation

Mitigation is the implementation of changes in systemic function based on analysis of lessons learned. Structural, strategic, and operational changes to the system seek to ensure more robust response and faster recovery in future events.

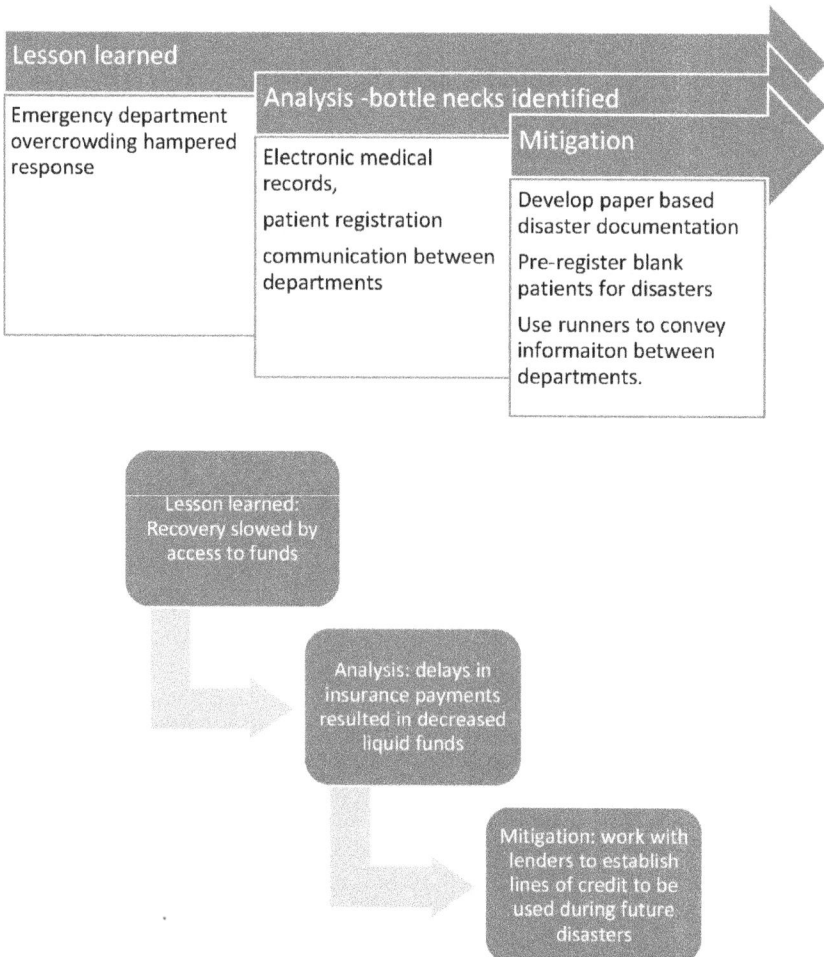

Lesson learned

Emergency department overcrowding hampered response

Analysis -bottle necks identified

Electronic medical records,

patient registration

communication between departments

Mitigation

Develop paper based disaster documentation

Pre-register blank patients for disasters

Use runners to convey informaiton between departments.

Lesson learned: Recovery slowed by access to funds

Analysis: delays in insurance payments resulted in decreased liquid funds

Mitigation: work with lenders to establish lines of credit to be used during future disasters

Examples of mitigation techniques:
Structural: building retro-fitting,
Human resources- reserve staffing
Material resources- stockpiling
Financial- lines of credit
Communication- use of radios, satellite phones
Administrative- established standard operating procedures and simplified disaster processes.

2.3.5 Preparedness

Preparedness represents the greatest period of the cycle longitudinally. Developing institutional plans, hazard vulnerability analysis with associated changes to plans, training, and licensing requirements all play key roles in the preparedness phase of the cycle. Additionally, given staff turnover, loss of institutional knowledge necessitates constant need for education.

3. Disaster medicine overview

3.1 Disaster medicine as a field

> 'a discipline resulting from the marriage of emergency medicine and disaster management'
>
> *- Gregory R. Ciottone, Disaster Medicine 2nd Edition [4]*

Disaster medicine as a field represents all the components of possible disasters. It is a clinical subspecialty encompassing a combination of medical aspects of care in disasters and elements of other non-medical fields [5]. Main topics of import are the crossover of emergency medical care and emergency management, health systems response to disasters, response structure from local to international, the concept of surge, and the pathology and treatment of individuals and populations during general and specific disasters. From a hospital and healthcare perspective, disaster medicine is most critical in the response, recovery and preparedness phases of the disaster cycle. Adjusting the system and provision of care during the surge of an event, continuing patient care, adapting to changes in the complex systems required in the provision of care, as well as working with the response organizations, are all concepts and practices within disaster medicine. In addition, the recovery of normal operations requires thoughtful and dedicated processes also within the fundamentals of disaster medicine. Lastly, the field of disaster medicine is fluid, requiring adaption to new threats as well as adoption of new understandings and best practices [6].

3.2 Anticipated pathology

The pathology of disaster events ranges from worsening of chronic disease, to trauma, to infectious diseases to event specific disease such as radiation sickness.

Examples of disaster related clinical pathology, its cause and its effect on hospital care.

- Trauma- any physical disruption, such as an act of violence, accidents, storms, earthquake all will increase trauma needs, often overwhelming hospitals.

- Infectious disease- a disaster itself, such as in an epidemic, or more commonly this is a result of the social disruption associated with the disaster. Increased rates of infections with displaced populations, loss of access to clean water or immunocompromise are all expected events. Community spread infection can overwhelm health systems.

- Disruption in chronic care- inability to access or provide care at the level of the community is an expectation in any major disaster. Interruptions in chronic care lead to complications and resultant accommodation by acute care hospitals.

- Psychological disease- sub-acute, acute, and chronic physiological consequences are all expected following a disaster event, as is worsening of baseline psychiatric disease. These patients can become high utilizers of health care services both primarily for the psychological needs and secondarily, its associated social, behavioral and somatic consequences.

3.3 Specialized needs

Some disaster events require specific training and specialist clinical care. Examples of these and associated specialized care needs are:

Radiologic emergencies

Toxic exposures

Bioterrorism

4. Elements of hospital function affected by disasters and security incidents

4.1 Reliance on the public and private sector

Healthcare delivery is contingent on many elements of normal social functioning. When a disaster disrupts government services, the private sector and the environment, hospital systems will have to adapt to continue with their mission.

Examples of healthcare's reliance on other parts of society:

Material resources from the private sector, From pharmaceuticals to gloves, hospitals need inputs from the private sector. This can be mitigated somewhat through stockpiling of supplies, however the practice of stockpiling is no longer a feasible model for many if not most healthcare institutions [7]. Some government programs may provide safety nets for supplies such as the strategic national stockpile in the United States.

Government services: Healthcare workers take the bus to work, they need their children to be in school in order to go to work, hospitals require police protection, waste services and utilities; some or all of which may be disrupted in a disaster.

4.2 Facilities

Any disaster event that causes physical damage to the hospital or healthcare facility will likely affect its ability to provide care. Examples include the obvious such as earthquakes and storms but also acts of violence and vandalism.

5. Healthcare workforce considerations

A major consideration with regards to health system functioning in a disaster, is that the healthcare workforce is affected by the disaster as much as the rest of society. The difference is that those in healthcare must still work when others are able to recover, and they share the emotional burden of others, bearing witness to their suffering. This can have a profound effect on wellbeing and efficacy in providing care. Worrying about loved ones while responding to a disaster event may have considerable consequences [8]. It is reasonable also to assume that despite their commitment and sense of duty to society, healthcare workers in a disaster who find themselves in the difficult situation of responding to their work or ensuring the safety and well being of their families are going to chose the latter.

5.1 Introduction

Functionality of the healthcare workforce in a disaster is a major consideration during all phases of the disaster cycle.

Few, if any, parts of society are going bear the burden of disasters more than healthcare workers and their families. Already dedicated to the wellbeing of the population, altruistic and hardworking, healthcare workers will be subject to conflicting responsibilities and seemingly insurmountable pressure. This untenable situation comes from three distinct consequences of the disaster. Increased workload, in the form of volume and acuity, emotional burden of being face to face with the tragedy of the disaster, familial responsibilities with less support than the rest of society, as they are still required to come to work. Additionally, as their work environment is also disrupted- for example supply shortages. Thus, their job is inherently more difficult. Hospital workers face even greater responsibilities with disruption of outpatient healthcare as these patients normally seen in clinics must now get their care in the hospital.

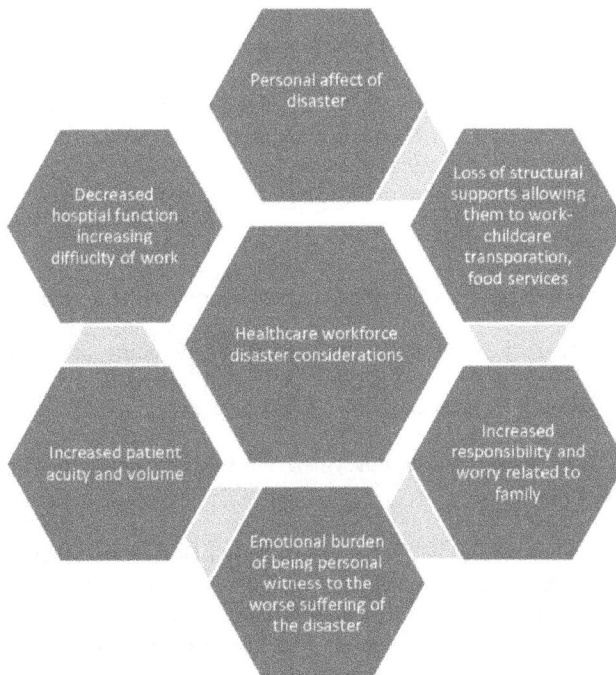

5.2 Healthcare workers disaster concerns

1. Healthcare workers are personally affected by the disaster the same as other members of society. Emotional distress, loss of housing, material resources, and health concerns. Death, injury, and illness of family without the ability to respond can be devastating.

2. Hospital function- despite the affects of structural destruction, materials shortage and increased patient volume, to name few pressures, healthcare workers at hospitals are expected to be present and preform.

3. Greater affects of social disruption- Healthcare workers rely on social services to support their work. Public transportation, elder and pet care, and childcare in the form of schools and after school activities. When these are disrupted the abilities healthcare workers on a practical and logisitional are diminished.

4. Healthcare workers have to preform major clinical problems in disasters: increased patient burden and acuity form the disaster itself, including those suffering from psychological affects and needing access to social services. Need to accommodate those who are unable to access care for acute and chronic health needs from disruption of outpatient healthcare, no changes in (non-disaster), healthcare needs of the their community.

5. Bearing witness to the worst of the suffering can have short and long term consequences on healthcare workers mental health [9].

5.3 Healthcare workforce resiliency

Maximizing healthcare worker performance in a disaster represents one of the greatest opportunities for disaster response and recovery. Some practical measures supporting healthcare workers include:

5.3.1 Healthcare worker family and household planning

Workers at all levels must have household planning that allows them to respond to work knowing that their family is safe and cared for. Any question family safety may result in failure to be present at work and/or suboptimal work performance.
Healthcare workers household safety plans should include:

• Household evacuation plans

• Agreements with family and friends to provide pet, child and elderly care.

• Two weeks of stocked material resources (food, medicine, comfort items)

• Backup utilities, communications and shelter plans.

5.3.2 Mutual aid agreements and health system collaboration for increased workforce resillancy

Establishing relationships with other healthcare institutions, with prearranged commitments of support can be crucial to an overwhelmed system.
Licensure planning allows for outside healthcare workers to provide care and support in a rapid manner. This involves rapid licensure and credentialing of out of system and/or out of the state or country healthcare workers.

5.4 Workforce wellbeing

Supporting workers wellbeing will increase efficacy and longevity. Examples of minimum support that should be planned for include:

- Private personal areas

- Food and hygiene

- Personal medicines,

- Scheduling to support rest and recovery

- Means for outside communication

- Structured and unstructured support of teambuilding and health before during and after a disaster

5.5 Labor unrest

A special disaster exists regarding healthcare workers and healthcare related labor disputes. These events can represent healthcare disasters in themselves and must be planned for accordingly. Hospital resiliency during these challenging situation can occur only with extensive management, collaboration and placing patient wellbeing before other priorities. Given the ethical challenges these situations represent all levels of the workforce maybe greatly affected [10].

6. Specific disaster and security considerations

6.1 Hazard vulnerability analysis

The all hazards approach means that planning can be adapted to any situation, but understanding the likelihood of occurrence and impact of specific disasters is paramount to good preparedness. Disaster planners use a hazard vulnerability analysis to quantify potential disaster events to their institution. This matrix uses a combination of the likelihood of an event will occur and severity of impact of the event to create a visual risk of disasters to the institution.

Example of a Hospital Hazard Vulnerability Matrix.

Low	**Likelihood of occurrence**			**High**
Low				Wind Storm
Impact to institutional function			Supply chain disruption	
		Plane crash		Multivehicle automotive crash
	Power Outage			
				Snow Strom
High	Earthquake			

6.2 Isolated violence

Acts of violence against healthcare workers, in or around healthcare institutions are common enough to have resulted in public outcry and public indifference. These events can have devastating effects on the individuals and institutions involved [11]. Promoting a culture of security including safety training (example active shooter training), freedom to disclose security concerns, engagement of all staff members in security planning and a weapons free environment all represent resiliency techniques [12].

6.3 Social unrest

This is an underestimated disaster with regards to its affect on healthcare. Social unrest from collective violence to political discord affect the mental and physical well being of the population and thus effect healthcare. General disaster planning should be sufficient, but messaging and communication to healthcare workers and the general population take on greater importance. The establishment and communication of the healthcare institutions as non-partisan and objective regarding the social unrest itself is paramount to continued function. Rumors increase anxiety and effect patients and clinicians alike and mis-information will fill any void in understanding. Communication of ability to provide care and overall function of healthcare delivery maybe a reassuring element in a time of crisis. Communication re-enforcing the positive public perception of healthcare as a benevolent social institution may also help healthcare delivery.

6.4 Inclement weather

With some notable exceptions (major storms), a major disruption in standards of care secondary to inclement weather represents a failure of planning and preparation. Preparing for events or seasons with enhanced materials stockpiling, health worker accommodations and transportation planning, fiscal considerations and planning for changes in burden of disease are all important issues enhancing event response.

6.5 Natural disasters

Severe natural disasters may poise the greatest disaster threat to peaceful societies. Events like earthquakes, major storms, and flooding can result in near or total societal disfunction. The affect on healthcare can be devastating. Mitigation of risks such as structural enhancement and pre-disaster evacuation, when possible, offer great promise with regard to resiliency. Acceptance of outside recourses, such as search and rescue, medical assistance teams, use of out of system healthcare and public health providers and evacuation teams all represent important response mechanisms.
Examples of support services:

- International search, rescue, and medical services teams

- Humanitarian aid organizations: such as the red cross and red crescent

- FEMA: Training, planning, expertise, logistical, material and financial support

- Unites States Health department of health and human services: Mobile medical teams (DMAT), healthcare workers supplementation, pharmacy (EPAP) and logistical support.

6.6 War and violent conflict

With its inherent effects on individuals and populations, including trauma, malnutrition, loss of chronic care and increased infectious disease potential, organized violent conflict has the greatest potential impact on population health. Health effects can last long after the conflict is resolved [13]. Mitigation and resilient response are challenging at the level of a hospital or even the broader health system. Reliance on outside resources, evacuation and the greater resources of military institutions may all provide support.

6.7 Pandemic

The COVID-19 pandemic has changed the nature of hospital and healthcare planning and response. While the all-hazards approach is still the dominant paradigm, increased emphasis has been placed on surge capacity, isolation and critical care. Additionally, planning at the regional and or country level has eclipsed planning on the health system and hospital level, apropos of the nature of the event. Another major change is regarding the manufacture and stockpiling of supplies [14]. Those essential for staff and patient safety and barriers to disease spread are no longer subject to just-in-time delivery model shortages.

7. Hospital and healthcare specific security concerns

7.1 Hospitals

Hospitals as soft targets of terrorism and in war is an old phenomenon and one that is a guaranteed to continue [15]. This is in part because of the added emotional and psychological importance of healthcare on society as well as the role healthcare facilities play in the broader aspects of social function. Additionally, the nature of healthcare delivery and its increased emotional implications, make it a more potent target for those interested in instilling fear and anger in the population.

7.2 Hospital

Hospital based security. Most hospitals have and should have significant baseline security. Bolstering this in the event of a disaster is key to avoiding violence affecting hospital care and patient's wellbeing.

7.3 Law

Law enforcement. Collaborations with law enforcement to increase supporting during and after a disaster event is also vital. It should be acknowledged that law enforcement priorities during a disaster are many and dynamic. While law enforcement support for healthcare should be encouraged and planned for, it should be accepted that it is not a guarantee. Additionally, in some circumstances of civil unrest the presence of law enforcement can be divisive.

7.4 Structural

Structural security. 'Lockdown,' a term used to prohibit unauthorized entry and exit from the hospital should be part of disaster planning and drills. Badges should be part and parcel of daily security measures and rigorously enforced during and after a disaster event or in times of high theat. Use of blocked entrances, unauthorizing of vehicles close to buildings, controlling of gatherings, screening for weapons and staff drilling for violent events should all be regular security principles employed in healthcare institutions.

8. The role of emergency medicine in disasters

Emergency medicine plays a critical role in disaster response and planning [16]. Understanding and appreciating its role and the importance of emergency medicine leadership in hospital planning are critical to hospital resiliency.

Issues affecting and mechanisms of resiliency regarding emergency medicine include:

8.1 Surge

Very few parts of healthcare ever need to undergo clinical surge, whereas in emergency medicine this is common and inevitable. The concept and practice of surge involves a paradigm of, and mechanisms for, flexibility. This impacts all areas of healthcare delivery, such as, the workforce, materials and environmental management and workflow [17].

8.2 Triage

Disaster triage relates not only to the need for choosing where and in what order to care for patients but also the limiting of resources when necessary. With regard to the order and location of care, emergency medicine with its understanding of diverse pathology, familiarity and relationship to other areas of the hospital, and focus on public health, trauma and infectious disease is ideally suited to triage. What is more is that during a disaster triage will become of greater importance as volumes of patients, some with no medical needs overwhelm the system. Limiting of care or Utilitarian theory referred to as 'maximize collective welfare' or to 'do the greatest good for the greatest numbers of people,' is another major component of disaster triage. The principle and practice of Utilitarian theory is part of emergency medicine training [18].

8.3 Access

Access to the health system. The emergency department is the most common way of accessing care in many health systems and it is likely to remain so during a disaster event. Utilizing this tried and established framework, with appropriate augmentation has many practical advantages.

Some Final thoughts

Hospitals and systems functioning at 110% of capacity have little chance of maximal response to a disaster.

Surge by definition requires systemic available capacity and flexibility.

Healthcare will be very limited following a disaster when hospitals and healthcare providers fail to plan.

Historically and predictably, workers rise to the occasion of disaster response, supporting their neighbors and communities in heroic ways.

Near complete absence of material reserves, now standard practice in American healthcare, is the weakest link in healthcare ability to respond to disasters .

In all things, begin as you intend to proceed. Robust planning and preparedness will lead to a robust response.

9. Conclusion

Resilient hospital and health system disaster response is dependent on under-standing the role hospitals play in disasters, their vulnerabilities and ways to support them. The importance of realizing hospital and health systems chang-ing roles during a disaster, its dependence on other parts of society and perhaps most importantly the challenges faced by its workforce drives disaster planning. Additionally, the threats to hospitals targeted or not, guides planning and response framework. Emergency medicine with its function as the entry way into the health system, understanding of diverse and all encompassing clinical pathology, practice involving surge and triage and its training in disaster medicine gives it a key role in disaster resilience for hospitals and health systems.

Conflict of interest

None.

Author details

Stephen C. Morris
University of Washington, Seattle, Washington, USA

*Address all correspondence to: stephenmorrismd@gmail.com

IntechOpen

References

[1] Heisler, M., Baker, E., & McKay, D. (2015). Attacks on health care in Syria—normalizing violations of medical neutrality?. *New England journal of medicine*, 373(26), 2489-2491.

[2] Cooper, C., & Swanson, N. (2002). Workplace violence in the health sector. *State of the art. Geneva: Organización Internacional de Trabajo, Organización Mundial de la Salud, Consejo Internacional de Enfermeras Internacional de Servicios Públicos*.

[3] Khan, H., Vasilescu, L. G., & Khan, A. (2008). Disaster management cycle-a theoretical approach. *Journal of Management and Marketing*, 6(1), 43-50.

[4] Ciottone, G. R., Biddinger, P. D., Darling, R. G., Fares, S., Keim, M. E., Molloy, M. S., & Suner, S. (Eds.). (2015). *Ciottone's disaster medicine*. Elsevier Health Sciences.

[5] Walsh, L., Subbarao, I., Gebbie, K., Schor, K. W., Lyznicki, J., Strauss-Riggs, K., ... & Hick, J. (2012). Core competencies for disaster medicine and public health. *Disaster Med Public Health Prep*, 6(1), 44-52.

[6] Arnold, J. L. (2002). Disaster medicine in the 21st century: future hazards, vulnerabilities, and risk. *Prehospital and Disaster Medicine*, 17(1), 3-11.

[7] Manos, A., Sattler, M., & Alukal, G. (2006). Make healthcare lean. *Quality progress*, 39(7), 24.

[8] Raveis, V. H., VanDevanter, N., Kovner, C. T., & Gershon, R. (2017). Enabling a disaster-resilient workforce: attending to individual stress and collective trauma. *Journal of Nursing Scholarship*, 49(6), 653-660.

[9] Zhang, G., Pfefferbaum, B., Narayanan, P., Lee, S., Thielman, S., & North, C. S. (2016). Psychiatric disorders after terrorist bombings among rescue workers and bombing survivors in Nairobi and rescue workers in Oklahoma City. *Annals of clinical psychiatry*.

[10] Chadwick, R., & Thompson, A. (2000). Professional ethics and labor disputes: Medicine and nursing in the United Kingdom. *Cambridge Q. Healthcare Ethics*, 9, 483.

[11] Lanctôt, N., & Guay, S. (2014). The aftermath of workplace violence among healthcare workers: A systematic literature review of the consequences. *Aggression and violent behavior*, 19(5), 492-501.

[12] Jacobs, L. M., & Burns, K. J. (2017). The Hartford consensus: survey of the public and healthcare professionals on active shooter events in hospitals. *Journal of the American College of Surgeons*, 225(3), 435-442.

[13] Ghobarah, H. A., Huth, P., & Russett, B. (2004). The post-war public health effects of civil conflict. *Social science & medicine*, 59(4), 869-884.

[14] Ranney, M. L., Griffeth, V., & Jha, A. K. (2020). Critical supply shortages—the need for ventilators and personal protective equipment during the Covid-19 pandemic. *New England Journal of Medicine*, 382(18), e41.

[15] De Cauwer, H., Somville, F., Sabbe, M., & Mortelmans, L. J. (2017). Hospitals: soft target for terrorism?. *Prehospital and disaster medicine*, 32(1), 94.

[16] der Heide, E. A. (2006). The importance of evidence-based disaster planning. *Annals of emergency medicine*, 47(1), 34-49.

[17] Kaji, A., Koenig, K. L., & Bey, T. (2006). Surge capacity for healthcare systems: a conceptual framework. *Academic Emergency Medicine*, *13*(11), 1157-1159.

[18] Sztajnkrycer, M. D., Madsen, B. E., & Báez, A. A. (2006). Unstable ethical plateaus and disaster triage. *Emergency Medicine Clinics*, *24*(3), 749-768.

Chapter 9

Impact of Climate Change on International Health Security: An Intersection of Complexity, Interdependence, and Urgency

Vikas Yellapu, Samuel Malan, Brandon Merkert,
Hetal Kharecha, Ambreen Alam and Stanislaw P. Stawicki

Abstract

Climate change (CC) can be defined as a long-term shift in global, continental, and/or local climate patterns. Although many equate CC to the rise in global temperatures, the issue is much more complicated and involves a large number of interconnected factors. Among some of the less discussed considerations of CC are its effects on a broad range of public health issues, including the emergence of novel infectious diseases, the encroachment of infectious disease vectors into previously unaffected geographic distributions, and crop failures resulting in threats of malnutrition and mass migration. This chapter will be devoted to key issues related to CC in the context of international health security (IHS).

Keywords: climate change, emerging infectious diseases, global warming, hunger, human migrations, invasive species

1. Introduction

Planet Earth is a highly complex and truly unique celestial body, fine-tuned to sustain life within a very narrow range of tolerances [1, 2]. Within this narrow band of environmental parameters, our civilization emerged over the past several thousand years. As we discovered ways in which to harness the energy stored within our planet, from burning wood, to coal, to petroleum products, we began to increasingly change the environment we live in [3, 4]. The resultant slow but persistent climate change (CC) is beginning to manifest itself across multiple domains of human existence, from rising sea levels, to wind disasters and forest fires, to the emergence of new invasive species [5–8]. This chapter will discuss the impact of CC on various domains of human health and well-being, with specific focus on their relationship to international health security (IHS). Given the vastness of this important topic area, our goal will be to provide an overview of the most pressing issues and most relevant subdomains (**Figure 1**). However, it is simply not feasible to cover this entire subject within a single book chapter, thus limiting the current manuscript to a bullet-point synopsis.

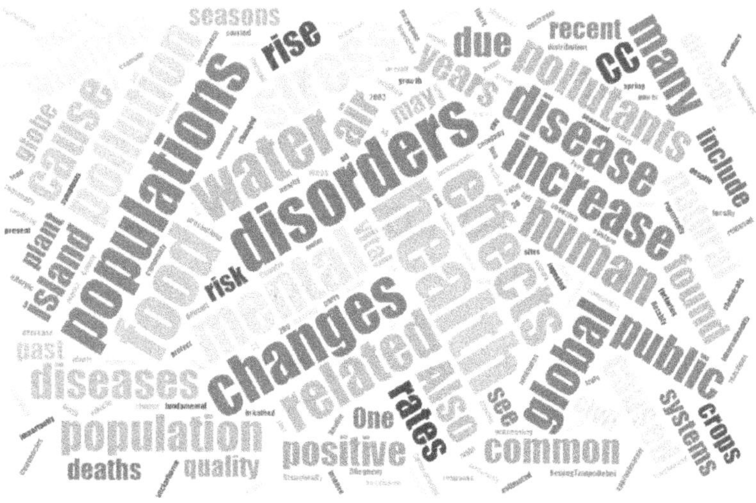

Figure 1.
Word cloud demonstrating the most common and dominant themes within this chapter. The highly complex nature of the issue of climate change and its relationship to human health is clearly evident.

2. Methodology

The current study constitutes a systematic review of the literature regarding the impact of climate change on human health and well-being. Relevant sources were identified using an exhaustive search strategy utilizing Google™ Scholar, PubMed, EBSCO, Bioline International, as well as any relevant cross-referenced articles and websites. Specific search terms included "climate change," "global warming," "invasive species," "emerging infectious diseases," "public health," "food security," "sea level change," "quality of life," and "vector-borne diseases." A total of 17,194,311 search results were subsequently narrowed down to 1,247 interdisciplinary full-text, English language articles directly relevant to our discussion. Further screening demonstrated 479 articles that directly address questions related to the interaction between climate change and human health and wellness. Of those, a final list of 266 definitive sources was derived.

3. Environmental pollution: air and water

The effects of air pollution on public health have become increasingly acute, heterogeneous, complex, and unpredictable [9–12]. In recent years, natural disasters such as wildfires and non-natural disasters such as human-made pollution have caused fundamental changes in air quality, leading to special measures and precautions deemed necessary to protect populations from air pollutants [13, 14]. Various effects of air pollution, both in the indoor and outdoor setting, on health include but are not limited to: asthma, chronic obstructive pulmonary disease (COPD), cardiovascular diseases, and an array of pulmonary malignancies [15–18]. Although naturally evolving changes in climate and temperature have some effect on air quality, direct human contribution to air pollution may play and even greater role [19, 20]. For example, humans are thought to be responsible for approximately 95% of all wildfires in California and in Mediterranean Europe [21, 22]. Wildfires diminish air quality by scorching thousands of acres of land – creating arid, dry, desert like soil, and a deterring vegetative and agricultural growth. Wildfires are only one example of many human activities that contribute to poor air quality [7, 23].

The continued growth of industrial activity, both in the United States and globally, has contributed to a sharp increase in air pollution, especially among the urban areas [24, 25]. This was accompanied by the general decline in measured air quality around the globe [26, 27]. Nowadays, air quality indexes are common in daily weather reporting, in addition to weather alerts for air quality standards [28, 29]. Despite the successful deployment of these largely descriptive and informative measures, much remains to be accomplished. For example, asthma amongst newborns and young children has increased sharply in the recent past [30].

Neville Island, PA is an inland island near Pittsburgh, PA where three major rivers meet, with at the apex of the city's heaviest population density [31]. The island houses more than 50 corporate industrial sites, coal processing facilities, and oil company foundries. The pollutants from these companies are ingested and breathed by the nearby population of the Allegheny County. During awareness campaigns in 2003, Neville Island was said to pollute river water with as many as 13 toxic chemicals hazardous to human health, reportedly released each night after the closing of the factories. Notably, the island is located just upstream to the County's major water treatment plant. Consequently, a broad range of pollutants (both airborne and non-airborne) find their way directly into the city water systems. Statistically, the County is among the highest in the nation for still births, childhood asthma, COPD, and pulmonary malignancy [31–33].

Historically, governmental regulations pertaining to air pollution tended to represent a more reactive (versus proactive) approach [34–36]. This is not universal, however. For example, the State of California has instituted aggressive standards for vehicle emission regulations. As a result, over a 20-year period there was a 65% decrease in reactive organic gases, and a 54% decrease in oxides of nitrogen [37]. Of importance, these positive changes occurred despite a 22% growth in population and a 38% increase in overall motor vehicle usage throughout the state [23]. There was an associated sharp and well-defined decrease in air pollution related breathing disorders among children. This included favorable changes in terms of asthma and bronchitis, with significant (21%-39%) reductions. With strict and appropriately enforced regulatory standards, a significant decline in adverse consequences of air pollution can clearly be achieved [23].

Still, environmental regulations are still poorly defined and/or neglected in many areas globally. Under such circumstances, countries like China experience a significant number of adverse health effects of air pollution, to the point of the issue becoming one of the most serious national public health threats [38]. Coal-burning power generation is among the leading culprits of air pollution in China [39]. The magnitude of coal-related pollution in China can be appreciated from recent data showing that in 2010, there were more than 10 million tons of fine particles (e.g., diameter under 2.5 μm) released in the Beijing-Tianjin-Hebei region alone [40]. The impact of such massive air pollution on human health and health security (locally, regionally, nationally, and internationally) is truly difficult to grasp. Even more importantly, it has been estimated that the pollution from the approximately 200 coal-fired power plants in the capital region of Beijing-Tianjin-Hebei may be associated with nearly 10,000 premature deaths and approximately 70,000 outpatient visits or hospitalizations during a single calendar year [40–42]. Despite the need for urgent reform at the global level, governments have been slow to act, including the recent unilateral (and hopefully temporary) withdrawal of the United States from the Paris Climate Pact [43].

4. Climate change: increase in allergens

One effect of global warming is an increase in allergens. Allergens can be associated with various respiratory diseases such as Asthma or allergic reactions such as hay fever. An increase in hay fever can be attributable to global temperature increases due to synergistic effects of atmospheric warming on the pollination season of plants [44]. The observed rise in the number of airborne allergens is directly proportional to the increase in pollen content of the air [45]. From human health perspective, it can be expected that allergic reactions, as well as their severity, may worsen over time. This may be further exacerbated by the declining air quality, both indoors and outdoors [46, 47].

The decrease in air quality is compounded by other factors such as smoking, diesel fuel utilization, and the generation of nitrogen dioxide [48–50]. Temperature fluctuations also lead to mold formation and propagation [51]. This can further decrease air quality and can cause intense allergic response in some people [52, 53]. Some other common allergies include ragweed allergy causing hay fever and poison ivy causing contact dermatitis. **Table 1** lists a set of common allergens. When an allergen enters the body, its presence leads to an immune response featuring the sensitization of mast cells [54, 55]. When the allergen enters the body repeatedly, it attaches to the specific antibodies on mast cells resulting in mast cell degranulation, which leads to the release of histamine and other inflammatory mediators [56, 57]. Associated symptoms may include commonly encountered reactions such as watery eyes, itching, sneezing, and nasal/sinus congestion. Pertinent to CC and global warming, it has been noted that patterns and distribution of common allergens typically present in different parts of the globe are changing [58]. The awareness and the ability to identify these patterns, coupled with modern mobile technology advances and point-of-care testing, will allow health-care providers to adequately prepare for the evolution and changing incidence of allergic reactions, especially in the context of preventive health measures and effective clinical management approaches [59–61].

5. Vector borne diseases and climate change

Another important aspect of the ongoing CC, and a source of indirect evidence for global warming, is the gradual evolution in disease vector distribution [8, 62]. An 'infectious vector' can be defined as any agent which carries and transmits an infectious pathogen into another living organism [63]. Many vector-borne diseases are characterized by a significant component of seasonality, and changing geographic distributions of vectors may significantly alter such seasonality [64, 65]. For example, higher rates of tick-borne diseases are seen during the spring to fall seasons in

Type of Allergen	Common Reaction to Allergen
Pollen	Seasonal allergies
Spores	Seasonal allergies, fungal infections
Dust mites	Asthma
Animal dander	Allergies
Drugs and insect venoms	Anaphylactic reaction

Table 1.
List of allergens and common reactions to those allergens.

eastern North America [66, 67]. With gradual temperature changes throughout the globe, we are more likely to see a change in the patterns of incidence of tick-borne illnesses [66, 67]. Moreover, novel tick-borne diseases have been on the rise, such as those carried by the Asian long-horned tick which has been found in the western hemisphere only in the past decade [66, 68]. Increased globalization and changes in environment due to global warming have been thought to increase the amount of tick-borne infections.

Some of the most common disease vectors are ticks and mosquitos. A summary of areas of prevalence and seasonality of tick- and mosquito-borne diseases are listed in **Tables 2** and **3**. When they reach sufficient magnitude, changes in environmental conditions are likely to disrupt the life cycle of various disease vectors and potentially alter the transmission of the diseases in question, including their geographic and seasonal distribution [66, 113].

Tick-Borne Illness	Areas of Prevalence	Predominant Months
Anaplasmosis [69]	USA: NY, MN, CT, RI, MD	May-October
Babesiosis [70]	USA: NY, NJ, MN, CT, MA, RI, WI	June-August
Colorado Tick Fever [71]	USA: WY, MT, UT, OR, CO, ID	May-July
Crimean-Congo [72, 73]	52 countries throughout Africa, Asia, Eastern Europe, and the Middle East	Spring-Summer
Ehrlichiosis [69]	USA: MO, OK, TN, AR, MD	May-September
Heartland Virus [74, 75]	USA: KS, OK, AR, MO, TN, KY, IN, GA, SC	May-September
Omsk Hemorrhagic Fever [76]	Western Siberia	May-June, August-September
Powassan Disease [77]	USA: MA, MN, NY, WI, NH, NJ, ME, ND, PA, TN, VT, VA, CT Canada: NB, QC, ON, NS, PE, AB, BC Russia: Primorsky Krai	May-November
Kyasanur Forest Disease [78]	India: Karnataka state and surrounding areas in the Western Ghats	January-May
Rocky Mountain Spotted Fever [79, 80]	USA: Contiguous states, >60% cases from NC, OK, AR, TN, and MO Canada, Mexico, Brazil, Columbia, Costa Rica, and Panama	April-September
Other Spotted Fevers [81–84]:		
African Tick-bite fever [81]	Sub-Saharan Africa and West Indies	November-April
Mediterranean spotted fever [82]	Africa, India, southern Europe, Middle East, Mediterranean	July-September
North Asian tick-borne rickettsiosis [83]	Armenia, central Asia, Siberia, Mongolia, China	April-May
Queensland tick Typhus [84]	Australia	June-November
Tularemia [85, 86]	North America, central Asia, Russia, the Nordic countries, the Balkans, and Japan USA: All states except HI, 50% of cases from AR, OK, and MO	April-October

Table 2.
Tick-Borne illnesses categorized by geographic distribution and yearly time range, focusing on the correlates of the highest prevalence of disease. United States and Canada jurisdictions are denoted using accepted two letter postal abbreviations.

Mosquito-Borne Illness	Areas of Prevalence	Predominant Months
Plasmodium Malariae [87, 88]	Africa and South Asia, Central and South America, the Caribbean, Southeast Asia, the Middle East, and Oceania	September-December
Dengue Virus [89, 90]	Americas, Eastern Mediterranean, South East Asia, and Western Pacific	March-August
Yellow Fever [91, 92]	47 countries throughout Africa (34) and Central and South America (13)	Africa: July-October South America: January-May
West Nile Virus [93–95]	Canada, USA-48 contiguous states, Europe, Africa, Middle East, Asia, India, Australia, Central America, Caribbean, South America	Northern Areas: July-October Southern Areas: Early months of the year
Zika Virus [8, 96, 97]	Africa, South East Asia, Oceania, Pacific Islands, South America, Central America, Caribbean, USA	Sporadic outbreaks Yap State: May 2007-June 2007 Pacific Islands: Late 2013- Early 2014 Americas 2015-2016: January 2016-July 2016
Bancroftian Filariasis [98]	72 countries throughout South East Asia, Sub-Saharan Africa, islands of Pacific, and selected areas in Latin America	Spring-Summer
Jamestown Canyon Virus [99, 100]	Canada: NL, QC, ON, MB, SK, NT USA: CT(1), LA(1), ME(2), MA(7), MI(1), MS(1), MT(1), NH(3), NJ(1), NY(4), NC(1), OH(2), OR(1), RI(1), TN(2), >50% MN(26) and WI(66)	April-September
Rift Valley Fever [101, 102]	Continental Africa, Yemen, Saudi Arabia, Madagascar, Comoros Islands, Mayotte	Outbreaks occur after heavy, prolonged rainfall
Chikungunya Virus [103, 104]	Africa, Asia, Indian Subcontinent	Northern Hemisphere: June–September Southern Hemisphere: October-March
Eastern Equine Encephalitis Virus [105, 106]	USA: AL (1), AR (1), CT (1), FL (13), GA (6), LA (2), ME (2), MD (1), MA (10), MI (7), MO (1), MT (1), NH (3), NJ (1), NY (8), NC (7), PA (1), RI (1), VT (2), VA (1), and WI (2)	April-October
Japanese Encephalitis Virus [107–109]	China, Japan, North Korea, South Korea, Australia, India, Pakistan, Russia, Singapore, Cambodia, Indonesia, Laos, Myanmar, India, Nepal, Malaysia, Philippines, Sri Lanka, Thailand, and Vietnam.	May-October
La Crosse Encephalitis Virus [110–112]	Upper Midwestern, mid-Atlantic, and Southeastern states	April-October

Table 3.
Mosquito-Borne illnesses organized by geographic area and seasonal time range characterized by the highest prevalence of disease. United States and Canada jurisdictions are denoted using accepted two letter postal abbreviations.

Countries around the globe are actively working on prevention measures intended to curb incidence levels of various vector borne diseases [114, 115]. Examples of preventative methods include application of insecticide spray, installing insecticide screens, improving sanitation methods, genetic modification

Infection	Source of contaminant
Escherichia coli 0157:H7	Undercooked beef
Giardiasis	Contaminated water
Cryptosporidiosis	Contaminated water
Campylobacteriosis	Undercooked poultry
Cyclosporiasis	Contaminated water or food
Listeriosis	Unpasteurized dairy products and deli meat
Salmonellosis	Undercooked poultry
Shigellosis	Contaminated water
Campylobacter	Undercooked poultry & other meats, contaminated water.
toxoplasmosis	Undercooked pork, lamb, shellfish, and venison.
Vibrio cholerae	Brackish and marine waters, or undercooked shellfish.

Table 4.
Common food and water borne illnesses and their source of contamination.

of vectors, as well as vector control through prophylactic treatment for travelers. Many countries are also intensifying awareness and education campaigns focusing on vector borne illness to help maintain prevention methods [114–117].

6. Food and water borne diseases

Global CC exerts impact on rainfall, humidity, length of growing season, and other environmental factors that are vital to the development of certain crops [118, 119]. Shifting environmental factors, along with the emergence of biofuels, are pushing food producers to implement various techniques that increase the yield of the crops [120]. One such method involves treating crops with antibiotics. However, unintended consequences of longer growing seasons and higher crop yields have resulted in greater frequency and intensity of food- and water-borne illness (**Table 4**) [121, 122]. Another way of coping with CC in terms of international food security is the introduction of insect-based, microbial/fungal-based, and laboratory-based food substitutes [123–129].

Of note, salmonella and campylobacter infections tend to be more common when the climate is warmer [130]. Relevant to human consumption, these bacteria have been shown to have higher growth rates at warmer temperatures during food preparation and storage [131], which in turn corroborates one possible relationship between CC and emerging human disease patterns.

The effect of CC on water borne diseases is equally important, yet it appears to be disproportionately neglected [132]. It is well known that precipitation can influence the transport and dissemination of infections, especially as it relates to existing water and sanitation systems [133]. More direct impact of the above can be seen during the increasingly more frequent coastal flooding as it relates to sea-level rise. Due to various factors, including human activity, water contamination exposes local populations to a variety of potential fecal-oral pathogens [134]. Indirect factors affecting the overall risk of water-borne infection propagation include changes in temperature and humidity, leading to alterations in pathogen lifecycle and survival, up to and including the creation of environments where new patterns of geographic disease spread emerge [135]. The effects of CC on water borne diseases, both indirect and direct, can be profound and unpredictable, mandating that dedicated scientific research efforts in this critically important area are increased.

7. Food security

Because agriculture relies heavily on the presence of favorable environmental parameters, any uncertainty related to agricultural conditions places food security into a state of flux and thus creates a potential threat to food sustainability and security for humans [136, 137]. Threats to food security are vast, diverse, and have increased sharply during the past three decades. Issues affecting food security involve agricultural, industrial, and climate-related components (e.g., from natural disasters to heavy pollution) [138, 139]. Protein-based food products from animal derived sources may contain significant antibiotic residue because antibiotics are increasingly utilized to maintain product viability and longevity during transport and distribution [140, 141]. Downstream effects of using antimicrobials in animal feed include various patterns of antibiotic resistance seen in both animals and humans who ingest animal-based food products [121, 142, 143]. Consequently, we are increasingly seeing emerging antibiotic resistance patterns that render many of our available therapeutics ineffective, leading to excess mortality [144–146]. Moreover, antibiotics have also leaked into water and food chains, creating complex and challenging matrices for the detection of their source of origin, which is vital to effective disease control [147, 148]. The importance of this complex phenomenon, in addition to introducing excess risk into the food chain and endangering the overall food security, is the potential for synergistic interactions between CC, emerging novel pathogens, and often unpredictable patterns of antimicrobial resistance [149–151]. As such, the confluence of the above factors is projected to result in significant food shortages, on *per capita* basis, by the year 2050. The attributable mortality may exceed 500,000 deaths around the globe [152]. Increased focus on ensuring food availability will be a crucial component of IHS in the future, and will be inextricably tied with the ongoing CC [7, 14]. Among promising sustainable growth strategies in this important area is the introduction and increasing implementation of the vertical farm concept [153]. Last, but not least, the gradual acidification of the oceans is beginning to affect the overall aquaculture and food chain sustainability, especially across the densely populated coastal areas that heavily rely on fish and other forms of seafood for ongoing food security [154–156]. Associated phenomena include harmful algal blooms which further damage aquatic ecosystems [157].

8. Flooding and flood-related events

Over the past several decades, floods have become a growing problem throughout the world [158, 159]. This has been especially problematic among low-lying areas of the planet, including large river deltas [160–164], and thought to be associated with rising sea levels [165–167]. It has been estimated that roughly 40-50% of environmental disasters are due to floods, and there is also a significant correlation between flooding and wind disasters [165–168]. From IHS perspective, floods may lead to drinking water contamination and associated increases in water borne and diarrheal diseases [169, 170]. It is therefore vital that we understand how to address and prevent deleterious public health consequences associated with flooding, inclusive of additional focus on a plethora of downstream effects of flooding on human populations [171–174].

In addition to immediate loss of life and property, there is a noticeable increase in diarrheal diseases, and studies suggest that there may also be an increased risk of all-cause mortality during the year following a flooding event [175, 176].

This troubling trend can be further exacerbated when flooding occurs in the presence of human overcrowding [176]. Of importance in this particular context, when planning and preparing for natural disasters it is important to understand the ecosystem of communicable diseases within the region and understand the vectors that may come into play. Effective management of flooding and subsequent post-event recovery requires proper sanitation, clean water supply at shelters/temporary housing for displaced individuals, as well as adequate control of disease vectors (e.g., rodents, mosquitoes) [177, 178]. Consequently, preventing contamination of standing water with mosquitoes should be priority during a flooding event [179, 180]. Governments planning for natural calamities, including floods and wind disasters, should ensure that appropriate supplies of clean water and food are readily available to large number of individuals. At the same time, it is also important to educate individuals on the importance of proper food and water preparation, through boiling, during any natural disaster that may potentially affect water supply [181–184].

9. Wildfires

Rising global temperature affects public health in urban and rural communities across the world [185]. In recent years urban heat waves have become more severe, which has corresponded with an increase in heat-attributable deaths during times of extreme summer temperatures [186]. In rural communities, phenomena such as dust storms and crop failures, along with invasive insect infestations and invasions, have increasingly appeared [187–193]. To make things worse, CC also creates an environment more prone to wildfires, which are affecting rural communities with increased frequency, and are progressively more common near more densely populated areas [7, 14, 194]. Human consequences of all of the above factors, especially when acting synergistically, will be both profound and difficult to calculate [7, 14]. As average global temperatures continue to rise it is imperative to quantify the burden that the health systems will face due to more severe heatwaves and wildfires [195].

Heatwaves are often defined as 2 or more consecutive days with temperatures above the 95th percentile for the summer [196, 197]. Relative risk of mortality increases during heatwaves in urban centers, particularly among elderly patients and patients with pre-existing cardiorespiratory conditions [198, 199]. This was demonstrated during an August 2003 heatwave in Europe, when heatwave-attributable mortality reached 14,800, the risk of out-of-hospital cardiac arrests increased by 14%, and hospitalizations significantly increased among asthma patients [200, 201]. Patients with pre-existing cardiorespiratory conditions were most at-risk for heat-related mortality [200, 201]. It is important to consider cardiovascular and respiratory conditions because they are among the most common pre-existing conditions within a progressively aging general population [202–205]. The specific physiologic processes causing increased mortality in patients with existing cardiovascular conditions during heatwaves are still poorly understood. However, it can be postulated that longer and more severe heatwaves place more strain on the cardiovascular system to maintain physiologic body temperatures via thermoregulation. Additionally, high temperatures are associated with elevated heart rate, increased blood viscosity from dehydration, and higher blood cholesterol levels. These factors together with sub-optimal electrolyte balance and reduced cerebral perfusion place higher demands on the cardiovascular system, which could exacerbate symptoms in vulnerable patients [206, 207].

Respiratory conditions on the other hand could be worsened because of lengthening frost-free periods and increasing levels of dusts and other pollutants in the urban atmosphere [208, 209]. This can be further exacerbated by the simultaneous presence of wildfires (e.g., California or Colorado, Summer 2020) [7, 14, 210, 211]. Evidence suggests that as carbon dioxide levels increase, ragweed (which is ubiquitous in urban communities) flowers earlier and produces 30-90% more pollen [212, 213]. By association, allergic sensitivity may lead to exacerbations of respiratory illness like asthma, but the phenomenon may have other synergistic components that are also directly or indirectly tied to CC [214].

Traditionally, rural communities have offered a relative escape from the smog and heat trapping environment of the city [215]. However, rising global temperatures are diminishing the air quality of rural communities by creating a dry landscape that is prone to wildfires and dust storms [216–218]. More specifically, particulate matter smaller than 2.5 um (PM2.5), carbon monoxide, nitrogen oxide, ozone precursors, and other harmful substances are released from wildfires, with various other components present within the cloud of a typical dust storm [154, 219, 220]. Of note, PM2.5 exposure during wildfires has been associated with increases in emergency department and hospital visits related to respiratory illnesses [221], with asthma exacerbations and wheezing in patients 65 and older having the greatest morbidity impact [222]. Evidence of cardiovascular and non-cardiopulmonary morbidity from particulate matter exposure is less consistent, with clear need for further research to better characterize any potential underlying associations [7].

10. Wind disasters

The number and severity of wind disasters appears to be increasing over the past two decades [168, 223, 224]. This connection between CC and increasing number and intensity of major hurricanes and other similar weather events is not fully understood [225], but more recent evidence does support a more causative effect [226, 227]. The current 2020 hurricane season in the United States is among the worst on historical record [228]. Its logistical impact is further compounded by the co-presence of the Novel Coronavirus pandemic [228]. Similar to flood disasters (which may also occur simultaneously), wind disasters and their aftermath may also have significant impact on life within the affected regions [229]. The impact of wind disasters on humans goes far beyond direct physical damage and bodily injuries [230]. Forced human migrations and post-traumatic stress add a massive component of complexity to the overall post-disaster recovery process [231–233]. Moreover, there seems to be an association between post-traumatic stress following wind disasters and the emergence of cardiovascular and other comorbid disease manifestations (or exacerbations) [231, 234]. Such longer-term manifestation appear to be more pronounced among members of underrepresented minorities, further highlighting issues of social and health-care inequity [231, 235, 236].

11. Climate change: effects on mental health and societal crises

Public health is influenced by a diverse collection of factors, many discussed in earlier sections of this chapter. One of the most under-appreciated factors is the effect of CC on mental health, both directly and indirectly, at both personal and societal levels [237, 238]. One of many subtle manifestations of societal distress is the proposed link between global warming, crop failures, and armed conflict [239, 240].

As a result, we begin to see greater incidence of mass migrations and refugee crises [241, 242]. An associated surge in mental disorders and stress related diseases is inextricably tied to such occurrences [243, 244]. Given the intersectionality of stress related disorders and their effect on the mental health of populations, it is not surprising that many are being pushed to their coping limits when faced with food insecurity, environmental pollution, increasing frequency of natural disasters, crops failures, and economic and political instability [245]. Moreover, long-term effects of such new global status quo are equally difficult to predict [246].

Large scale human migrations due to natural disasters, conflict, famine, or political and economic instability, have been associated with mental health and stress related illnesses across the globe [247–249]. All population segments are affected, from rich to poor, from urban to rural, from young to old, without exception [250–252]. Exposures to potentially traumatic events, regardless of the exact nature of the event, are known to cause an increased risk for mental disorders including post-traumatic stress disorder (PTSD) [253–255]. Associated downstream consequences may include increased incidence of depression and increased suicide rates [256].

Significant proportion of the world's population does not have sufficient access to mental health support, including both high income regions (HIRs) and low-and-middle-income regions (LMIRs) [257–260]. Individuals from regions affected by CC (and secondary phenomena related to CC) may find themselves experiencing a myriad of stressors affecting mental health and resulting in various stress related diseases (including substance abuse) [245]. At the personal level, a number of different approaches can be used to effectively manage behavioral health symptoms, including cognitive behavioral therapies, medical-based treatments, as well as short- and long-term coping management therapies, with generally positive outcomes [261, 262]. At the societal level, public health education regarding mental health and wellness is of great importance [263–265]. Of course, governments and societies must continue to curb and address situations that contribute to ongoing stress and mental health related disorders. This focus in particular is critical to stabilizing populations affected most by CC and related crises [266].

12. Conclusion

Global climate change creates a multifactorial, highly complex matrix of direct and indirect effects that have the potential to threaten international health security. The many domains that synergistically affect human health in the context of CC include environmental pollution, the emergence of invasive species and novel pathogens, food security, wildfires, and a broad range of destructive weather events. Of course, the complete list is much more extensive, and beyond the scope of the current chapter. In summary, the global community must come together to more effectively and more systematically address issues associated with the ongoing CC and its many direct and indirect effects. To pretend that CC "does not exist" will be, simply said, too costly.

Author details

Vikas Yellapu[1], Samuel Malan[3], Brandon Merkert[3], Hetal Kharecha[4], Ambreen Alam[2] and Stanislaw P. Stawicki[2*]

1 Department of Internal Medicine, Richard A. Anderson Campus, St. Luke's University Health Network, Easton, PA, USA

2 Department of Research and Innovation, University Campus, St. Luke's University Health Network, Bethlehem, PA, USA

3 Medical School of Temple University/St. Luke's University Health Network, University Hospital Campus, Bethlehem, PA, USA

4 St. Luke's Physician Group, Bethlehem, PA, USA

*Address all correspondence to: stawicki.ace@gmail.com

IntechOpen

References

[1] VandenBerghe, L., *The Significance of Humans in the Universe: The Purpose and Meaning of Life*. 2019: AuthorHouse.

[2] Eldredge, N., *The miner's canary: Unraveling the mysteries of extinction*. Vol. 13. 1994: Princeton University Press.

[3] Malm, A., *Fossil capital: The rise of steam power and the roots of global warming*. 2016: Verso Books.

[4] Herzog, H., E. Drake, and E. Adams, *CO2 capture, reuse, and storage technologies for mitigating global climate change*. A white paper, 1997: p. 1-70.

[5] Giorgi, F. and P. Lionello, *Climate change projections for the Mediterranean region*. Global and planetary change, 2008. **63**(2-3): p. 90-104.

[6] Harvey, B.J., *Human-caused climate change is now a key driver of forest fire activity in the western United States*. Proceedings of the National Academy of Sciences, 2016. **113**(42): p. 11649-11650.

[7] Le, N.K., et al., *International Health Security: A Summative Assessment by ACAIM Consensus Group*, in *Contemporary Developments and Perspectives in International Health Security-Volume 1*. 2020, IntechOpen.

[8] Sikka, V., et al., *The emergence of Zika virus as a global health security threat: a review and a consensus statement of the INDUSEM Joint Working Group (JWG)*. Journal of global infectious diseases, 2016. **8**(1): p. 3.

[9] Gao, J., et al., *Haze, public health and mitigation measures in China: A review of the current evidence for further policy response*. Science of the Total Environment, 2017. **578**: p. 148-157.

[10] de Prado Bert, P., et al., *The effects of air pollution on the brain: a review of studies interfacing environmental epidemiology and neuroimaging*. Current environmental health reports, 2018. **5**(3): p. 351-364.

[11] Duan, R.-R., K. Hao, and T. Yang, *Air pollution and chronic obstructive pulmonary disease*. Chronic Diseases and Translational Medicine, 2020.

[12] Klepac, P., et al., *Ambient air pollution and pregnancy outcomes: A comprehensive review and identification of environmental public health challenges*. Environmental research, 2018. **167**: p. 144-159.

[13] Akhtar, R. and C. Palagiano, *Climate Change and Air Pollution: An Introduction*, in *Climate Change and Air Pollution*. 2018, Springer. p. 3-8.

[14] Le, N.K., et al., *What's new in Academic International Medicine? International health security agenda– Expanded and re-defined*. International Journal of Academic Medicine, 2020. **6**(3): p. 163.

[15] Dickey, J.H., *Selected topics related to occupational exposures Part VII. Air pollution: Overview of sources and health effects*. Disease-a-month, 2000. **46**(9): p. 566-589.

[16] Association, A.L., *Urban air pollution and health inequities: a workshop report*. Environmental Health Perspectives, 2001. **109**(suppl 3): p. 357-374.

[17] Tham, K.W., *Indoor air quality and its effects on humans—A review of challenges and developments in the last 30 years*. Energy and Buildings, 2016. **130**: p. 637-650.

[18] Jones, A.P., *Indoor air quality and health*. Atmospheric environment, 1999. **33**(28): p. 4535-4564.

[19] Kim, K.-H., E. Kabir, and S. Ara Jahan, *A review of the consequences of*

global climate change on human health. Journal of Environmental Science and Health, Part C, 2014. **32**(3): p. 299-318.

[20] Leggett, J.A., *Evolving Assessments of Human and Natural Contributions to Climate Change*. 2018: Congressional Research Service.

[21] Vilar, L., et al., *Modeling temporal changes in human-caused wildfires in Mediterranean Europe based on land use-land cover interfaces.* Forest Ecology and Management, 2016. **378**: p. 68-78.

[22] Course, A.C., *Cannabis in California—*.

[23] Gilliland, F., et al., *The effects of policy-driven air quality improvements on children's respiratory health.* Research Reports: Health Effects Institute, 2017. **2017**.

[24] Hogrefe, C., et al., *Simulating changes in regional air pollution over the eastern United States due to changes in global and regional climate and emissions.* Journal of Geophysical Research: Atmospheres, 2004. **109**(D22).

[25] Faiz, A., *Automotive air pollution: Issues and options for developing countries.* Vol. 492. 1990: World Bank Publications.

[26] Molina, M.J. and L.T. Molina, *Megacities and atmospheric pollution.* Journal of the Air & Waste Management Association, 2004. **54**(6): p. 644-680.

[27] Fenger, J., *Urban air quality.* Atmospheric environment, 1999. 33(29): p. 4877-4900.

[28] Dabberdt, W.F., et al., *Meteorological research needs for improved air quality forecasting: Report of the 11th Prospectus Development Team of the US Weather Research Program.* Bulletin of the American Meteorological Society, 2004. 85(4): p. 563-586.

[29] Elsom, D., *Smog alert: managing urban air quality*. 2014: Routledge.

[30] Kim, J.J., *Ambient air pollution: health hazards to children.* Pediatrics, 2004. **114**(6): p. 1699-1707.

[31] Tatone, G. and D. Holland, *Neville Island.* Images of America. 2008, Charleston, SC: Arcadia Pub. 127 p.

[32] Gilliland, F., et al., *The Effects of Policy-Driven Air Quality Improvements on Children's Respiratory Health.* Res Rep Health Eff Inst, 2017(190): p. 1-75.

[33] Goodell, M.Z., *The Island : Neville island in the 1960s: an eden on the Ohio.* 2014, Bloomington, IN: ArchwayPub. pages cm.

[34] Cramer, J.C., *Population growth and local air pollution: methods, models, and results.* Population and Development Review, 2002. **28**: p. 22-52.

[35] Chen, T.-M., et al., *Outdoor air pollution: overview and historical perspective.* The American journal of the medical sciences, 2007. **333**(4): p. 230-234.

[36] Handl, G., *International efforts to protect the global atmosphere: A case of too little, too late.* Eur. J. Int'l L., 1990. **1**: p. 250.

[37] Lurmann, F., E. Avol, and F. Gilliland, *Emissions reduction policies and recent trends in Southern California's ambient air quality.* Journal of the Air & Waste Management Association, 2015. **65**(3): p. 324-335.

[38] McMichael, A.J., *The urban environment and health in a world of increasing globalization: issues for developing countries.* Bulletin of the world Health Organization, 2000. **78**: p. 1117-1126.

[39] Wei, Y., et al., *Uncovering the culprits of air pollution: Evidence from China's*

economic sectors and regional heterogeneities. Journal of Cleaner Production, 2018. **171**: p. 1481-1493.

[40] Huang, C., et al., *Air Pollution Prevention and Control Policy in China.* Adv Exp Med Biol, 2017. **1017**: p. 243-261.

[41] Ahlers, C.D., *Wood Burning, Air Pollution, and Climate Change.* Envtl. L., 2016. **46**: p. 49.

[42] Guo, X., et al., *Air quality improvement and health benefit of PM 2.5 reduction from the coal cap policy in the Beijing–Tianjin–Hebei (BTH) region, China.* Environmental Science and Pollution Research, 2018. **25**(32): p. 32709-32720.

[43] Rhodes, C.J., *US withdrawal from the COP21 Paris climate change agreement, and its possible implications.* Science Progress, 2017. **100**(4): p. 411-419.

[44] Schmidt, C.W., *Pollen overload: seasonal allergies in a changing climate.* 2016, National Institute of Environmental Health Sciences.

[45] Hyde, H., *Atmospheric pollen and spores in relation to allergy. I.* Clinical & Experimental Allergy, 1972. **2**(2): p. 153-179.

[46] Kim, K.-H., S.A. Jahan, and E. Kabir, *A review on human health perspective of air pollution with respect to allergies and asthma.* Environment international, 2013. **59**: p. 41-52.

[47] Nazaroff, W.W., *Exploring the consequences of climate change for indoor air quality.* Environmental Research Letters, 2013. **8**(1): p. 015022.

[48] Liaquat, A., et al., *Potential emissions reduction in road transport sector using biofuel in developing countries.* Atmospheric Environment, 2010. **44**(32): p. 3869-3877.

[49] Yang, W., G. Yuan, and J. Han, *Is China's air pollution control policy effective? Evidence from Yangtze River Delta cities.* Journal of Cleaner Production, 2019. **220**: p. 110-133.

[50] Allen, D.T., *Emissions from oil and gas operations in the United States and their air quality implications.* Journal of the Air & Waste Management Association, 2016. **66**(6): p. 549-575.

[51] Northolt, M.D. and L.B. Bullerman, *Prevention of mold growth and toxin production through control of environmental conditions.* Journal of Food Protection, 1982. **45**(6): p. 519-526.

[52] Bernard, S.M., et al., *The potential impacts of climate variability and change on air pollution-related health effects in the United States.* Environmental health perspectives, 2001. **109**(suppl 2): p. 199-209.

[53] Singh, J., *Toxic moulds and indoor air quality.* Indoor and Built Environment, 2005. **14**(3-4): p. 229-234.

[54] Ma, H. and P.T. Kovanen, *IgE-dependent generation of foam cells: an immune mechanism involving degranulation of sensitized mast cells with resultant uptake of LDL by macrophages.* Arteriosclerosis, thrombosis, and vascular biology, 1995. **15**(6): p. 811-819.

[55] Lichtenstein, L.M., *Allergy and the immune system.* Scientific American, 1993. **269**(3): p. 116-124.

[56] Hellman, L.T., et al., *Tracing the origins of IgE, mast cells, and allergies by studies of wild animals.* Frontiers in immunology, 2017. **8**: p. 1749.

[57] Mandhane, S.N., J.H. Shah, and R. Thennati, *Allergic rhinitis: an update on disease, present treatments and future prospects.* International immunopharmacology, 2011. **11**(11): p. 1646-1662.

[58] Davies, J., *Grass pollen allergens globally: the contribution of subtropical grasses to burden of allergic respiratory diseases.* Clinical & Experimental Allergy, 2014. **44**(6): p. 790-801.

[59] Shea, K.M., et al., *Climate change and allergic disease.* Journal of allergy and clinical immunology, 2008. **122**(3): p. 443-453.

[60] Matricardi, P.M., et al., *The role of mobile health technologies in allergy care: An EAACI position paper.* Allergy, 2020. **75**(2): p. 259-272.

[61] Stawicki, S.P., et al., *Academic college of emergency experts in India's INDO-US Joint Working Group and OPUS12 foundation consensus statement on creating a coordinated, multi-disciplinary, patient-centered, global point-of-care biomarker discovery network.* International journal of critical illness and injury science, 2014. **4**(3): p. 200.

[62] Khasnis, A.A. and M.D. Nettleman, *Global warming and infectious disease.* Archives of medical research, 2005. **36**(6): p. 689-696.

[63] Sarwar, M., *Insect vectors involving in mechanical transmission of human pathogens for serious diseases.* Int J Bioinform Biomed Eng, 2015. **1**(3): p. 300-306.

[64] Churakov, M., et al., *Spatio-temporal dynamics of dengue in Brazil: Seasonal travelling waves and determinants of regional synchrony.* PLoS neglected tropical diseases, 2019. **13**(4): p. e0007012.

[65] Campbell-Lendrum, D., et al., *Climate change and vector-borne diseases: what are the implications for public health research and policy?* Philosophical Transactions of the Royal Society B: Biological Sciences, 2015. **370**(1665): p. 20130552.

[66] Gray, J., et al., *Effects of climate change on ticks and tick-borne diseases in Europe.* Interdisciplinary perspectives on infectious diseases, 2009. **2009**.

[67] Dantas-Torres, F., *Climate change, biodiversity, ticks and tick-borne diseases: the butterfly effect.* International Journal for Parasitology: parasites and wildlife, 2015. **4**(3): p. 452-461.

[68] Ergünay, K., *Revisiting new tick-associated viruses: what comes next?* Future Virology, 2020. **15**(1): p. 19-33.

[69] DEMMA, L.J., et al., *EPIDEMIOLOGY OF HUMAN EHRLICHIOSIS AND ANAPLASMOSIS IN THE UNITED STATES, 2001-2002.* The American Journal of Tropical Medicine and Hygiene, 2005. **73**(2): p. 400-409.

[70] *Babesiosis surveillance - 18 States, 2011.* MMWR Morb Mortal Wkly Rep, 2012. **61**(27): p. 505-9.

[71] Yendell, S.J., M. Fischer, and J.E. Staples, *Colorado tick fever in the United States, 2002-2012.* Vector-Borne and Zoonotic Diseases, 2015. **15**(5): p. 311-316.

[72] Appannanavar, S.B. and B. Mishra, *An update on Crimean Congo hemorrhagic fever.* Journal of global infectious diseases, 2011. **3**(3): p. 285.

[73] Bente, D.A., et al., *Crimean-Congo hemorrhagic fever: history, epidemiology, pathogenesis, clinical syndrome and genetic diversity.* Antiviral research, 2013. **100**(1): p. 159-189.

[74] Brault, A.C., et al., *Heartland virus epidemiology, vector association, and disease potential.* Viruses, 2018. **10**(9): p. 498.

[75] Pastula, D.M., et al., *Notes from the field: Heartland virus disease-United States, 2012-2013.* MMWR. Morbidity

and mortality weekly report, 2014.
63(12): p. 270-271.

[76] Gritsun, T., P. Nuttall, and E.A.
Gould, *Tick-borne flaviviruses*, in
Advances in virus research. 2003, Elsevier.
p. 317-371.

[77] Kemenesi, G. and K. Bányai,
*Tick-borne flaviviruses, with a focus on
powassan virus*. Clinical microbiology
reviews, 2018. **32**(1).

[78] Pattnaik, P., *Kyasanur forest disease:
an epidemiological view in India*. Reviews
in medical virology, 2006. **16**(3):
p. 151-165.

[79] NORD. *Rocky Mountain Spotted
Fever*. 2020 October 8, 2020]; Available
from: https://rarediseases.org/rare-
diseases/
rocky-mountain-spotted-fever/.

[80] Phillips, J., *Rocky Mountain spotted
fever*. Workplace Health & Safety, 2017.
65(1): p. 48-48.

[81] Jensenius, M., et al., *African tick bite
fever*. The Lancet infectious diseases,
2003. **3**(9): p. 557-564.

[82] Rovery, C. and D. Raoult,
Mediterranean spotted fever. Infectious
disease clinics of North America, 2008.
22(3): p. 515-530.

[83] Parola, P., et al., *Update on tick-
borne rickettsioses around the world:
a geographic approach*. Clinical
microbiology reviews, 2013. **26**(4):
p. 657-702.

[84] Stewart, A., et al., *Rickettsia
australis and Queensland tick typhus: a
rickettsial spotted fever group infection in
Australia*. The American journal of
tropical medicine and hygiene, 2017.
97(1): p. 24-29.

[85] Harik, N.S., *Tularemia:
epidemiology, diagnosis, and treatment.*

Pediatric Annals, 2013. **42**(7):
p. 288-292.

[86] Gürcan, Ş., *Epidemiology of
tularemia*. Balkan medical journal, 2014.
31(1): p. 3.

[87] Mueller, I., P.A. Zimmerman, and
J.C. Reeder, *Plasmodium malariae and
Plasmodium ovale–the 'bashful' malaria
parasites*. Trends in parasitology, 2007.
23(6): p. 278-283.

[88] Collins, W.E. and G.M. Jeffery,
*Plasmodium malariae: parasite and
disease*. Clinical microbiology reviews,
2007. **20**(4): p. 579-592.

[89] Hopp, M.J. and J.A. Foley, *Global-
scale relationships between climate and the
dengue fever vector, Aedes aegypti*.
Climatic change, 2001. **48**(2-3):
p. 441-463.

[90] Hopp, M.J. and J.A. Foley,
*Worldwide fluctuations in dengue fever
cases related to climate variability*.
Climate Research, 2003. **25**(1): p. 85-94.

[91] Christophers, S.R., *Aedes aegypti: the
yellow fever mosquito*. 1960: CUP
Archive.

[92] Brunette, G.W., *CDC Yellow Book
2018: health information for international
travel*. 2017: Oxford University Press.

[93] Rossi, S.L., T.M. Ross, and J.D.
Evans, *West nile virus*. Clinics in
laboratory medicine, 2010. **30**(1):
p. 47-65.

[94] Hayes, E.B., et al., *Epidemiology and
transmission dynamics of West Nile virus
disease*. Emerging infectious diseases,
2005. **11**(8): p. 1167.

[95] Campbell, G.L., et al., *West nile
virus*. The Lancet infectious diseases,
2002. **2**(9): p. 519-529.

[96] Hills, S.L., M. Fischer, and L.R.
Petersen, *Epidemiology of Zika virus*

infection. The Journal of Infectious Diseases, 2017. **216**(suppl_10): p. S868-S874.

[97] Duffy, M.R., et al., *Zika virus outbreak on Yap Island, federated states of Micronesia.* New England Journal of Medicine, 2009. **360**(24): p. 2536-2543.

[98] Zulfiqar, H., A. Waheed, and A. Malik, *Bancroftian Filariasis*, in *StatPearls [Internet]*. 2019, StatPearls Publishing.

[99] Grimstad, P.R., et al., *Jamestown Canyon virus (California serogroup) is the etiologic agent of widespread infection in Michigan humans.* The American journal of tropical medicine and hygiene, 1986. **35**(2): p. 376-386.

[100] Pastula, D.M., et al., *Jamestown Canyon virus disease in the United States—2000-2013.* The American journal of tropical medicine and hygiene, 2015. **93**(2): p. 384-389.

[101] Linthicum, K.J., et al., *Climate and satellite indicators to forecast Rift Valley fever epidemics in Kenya.* Science, 1999. **285**(5426): p. 397-400.

[102] Anyamba, A., et al., *Prediction of a Rift Valley fever outbreak.* Proceedings of the National Academy of Sciences, 2009. **106**(3): p. 955-959.

[103] Jupp, P. and B. McIntosh, *Chikungunya virus disease.* The arboviruses: epidemiology and ecology, 1988. **2**: p. 137-157.

[104] Schwartz, O. and M.L. Albert, *Biology and pathogenesis of chikungunya virus.* Nature Reviews Microbiology, 2010. **8**(7): p. 491-500.

[105] Armstrong, P.M. and T.G. Andreadis, *Eastern equine encephalitis virus—old enemy, new threat.* N Engl J Med, 2013. **368**(18): p. 1670-3.

[106] Armstrong, P.M. and T.G. Andreadis, *Eastern equine encephalitis*

virus in mosquitoes and their role as bridge vectors. Emerging infectious diseases, 2010. **16**(12): p. 1869.

[107] Endy, T. and A. Nisalak, *Japanese encephalitis virus: ecology and epidemiology*, in *Japanese encephalitis and West Nile viruses*. 2002, Springer. p. 11-48.

[108] Solomon, T., et al., *Origin and evolution of Japanese encephalitis virus in southeast Asia.* Journal of virology, 2003. **77**(5): p. 3091-3098.

[109] Solomon, T., et al., *Poliomyelitis-like illness due to Japanese encephalitis virus.* The Lancet, 1998. **351**(9109): p. 1094-1097.

[110] Burkot, T. and G. Defollart, *Bloodmeal sources of Aedes triseriatus and Aedes vexans in a southern Wisconsin forest endemic for La Crosse encephalitis virus.* The American Journal of Tropical Medicine and Hygiene, 1982. **31**(2): p. 376-381.

[111] Nasci, R.S., et al., *La Crosse encephalitis virus habitat associations in Nicholas County, West Virginia.* Journal of medical entomology, 2000. **37**(4): p. 559-570.

[112] Lee, J.-H., et al., *Simultaneous detection of three mosquito-borne encephalitis viruses (eastern equine, La Crosse, and St. Louis) with a single-tube multiplex reverse transcriptase polymerase chain reaction assay.* Journal of the American Mosquito Control Association-Mosquito News, 2002. **18**(1): p. 26-31.

[113] Wu, X., et al., *Impact of climate change on human infectious diseases: Empirical evidence and human adaptation.* Environment international, 2016. **86**: p. 14-23.

[114] Alphey, L., et al., *Sterile-insect methods for control of mosquito-borne diseases: an analysis.* Vector-Borne and

Zoonotic Diseases, 2010. **10**(3): p. 295-311.

[115] Gubler, D.J., et al., *Climate variability and change in the United States: potential impacts on vector-and rodent-borne diseases.* Environmental health perspectives, 2001. **109**(suppl 2): p. 223-233.

[116] Yasuoka, J., et al., *Impact of education on knowledge, agricultural practices, and community actions for mosquito control and mosquito-borne disease prevention in rice ecosystems in Sri Lanka.* The American journal of tropical medicine and hygiene, 2006. **74**(6): p. 1034-1042.

[117] Tolle, M.A., *Mosquito-borne diseases.* Current problems in pediatric and adolescent health care, 2009. **39**(4): p. 97-140.

[118] Ali, S., et al., *Climate Change and Its Impact on the Yield of Major Food Crops: Evidence from Pakistan.* Foods (Basel, Switzerland), 2017. **6**(6): p. 39.

[119] Olesen, J.E. and M. Bindi, *Consequences of climate change for European agricultural productivity, land use and policy.* European journal of agronomy, 2002. **16**(4): p. 239-262.

[120] Rathmann, R., A. Szklo, and R. Schaeffer, *Land use competition for production of food and liquid biofuels: An analysis of the arguments in the current debate.* Renewable Energy, 2010. **35**(1): p. 14-22.

[121] Yellapu, V., et al., *Key factors in antibiotic resistance.* Journal of Global Infectious Diseases, 2019. **11**(4): p. 163.

[122] Marshall, B.M. and S.B. Levy, *Food animals and antimicrobials: impacts on human health.* Clinical microbiology reviews, 2011. **24**(4): p. 718-733.

[123] Dossey, A., J. Tatum, and W. McGill, *Modern insect-based food industry: current status, insect processing technology, and recommendations moving forward,* in *Insects as sustainable food ingredients.* 2016, Elsevier. p. 113-152.

[124] Guo, Y., et al., *Nano-bacterial cellulose/soy protein isolate complex gel as fat substitutes in ice cream model.* Carbohydrate polymers, 2018. **198**: p. 620-630.

[125] Hashempour-Baltork, F., et al., *Mycoproteins as safe meat substitutes.* Journal of Cleaner Production, 2020. **253**: p. 119958.

[126] Newmark, P., *Meat substitutes: Fungal food.* Nature, 1980. **287**(5777): p. 6-6.

[127] Mayhall, T.A., *The Meat of the Matter: Regulating a Laboratory-Grown Alternative.* Food & Drug LJ, 2019. **74**: p. 151.

[128] Mouat, M.J., R. Prince, and M.M. Roche, *Making value out of ethics: The emerging economic geography of lab-grown meat and other animal-free food products.* Economic Geography, 2019. **95**(2): p. 136-158.

[129] Joffre, T. *Starving Yemenis find food source in massive locust outbreak.* 2019 Oct 28, 2020]; Available from: https://www.jpost.com/middle-east/starving-yemenis-find-food-source-in-massive-locust-outbreak-591426.

[130] Bryan, F.L. and M.P. Doyle, *Health Risks and Consequences of Salmonella and Campylobacter jejuni in Raw Poultry.* Journal of Food Protection, 1995. **58**(3): p. 326-344.

[131] White, P., A. Baker, and W. James, *Strategies to control Salmonella and Campylobacter in raw poultry products.* Revue scientifique et technique-Office international des épizooties, 1997. **16**: p. 525-541.

[132] Cissé, G., *Food-borne and water-borne diseases under climate change in*

low-and middle-income countries: Further efforts needed for reducing environmental health exposure risks. Acta tropica, 2019. **194**: p. 181-188.

[133] Cissé, G., et al., *Vulnerabilities of water and sanitation at households and community levels in face of climate variability and change: trends from historical climate time series in a West African medium-sized town.* International Journal of Global Environmental Issues, 2016. **15**(1-2): p. 81-99.

[134] Walker, J., *The influence of climate change on waterborne disease and Legionella: a review.* Perspectives in public health, 2018. **138**(5): p. 282-286.

[135] Wu, X., et al., *Impact of global change on transmission of human infectious diseases.* Science China Earth Sciences, 2014. **57**(2): p. 189-203.

[136] Ziervogel, G., et al., *Climate variability and change: Implications for household food security.* Assessment of Impacts and Adaptations to Climate Change (AIACC): Washington, DC, USA, 2006.

[137] Reddy, P.P., *Climate resilient agriculture for ensuring food security.* Vol. 373. 2015: Springer.

[138] Lioubimtseva, E. and G.M. Henebry, *Climate and environmental change in arid Central Asia: Impacts, vulnerability, and adaptations.* Journal of Arid Environments, 2009. **73**(11): p. 963-977.

[139] Edame, G.E., et al., *Climate change, food security and agricultural productivity in Africa: Issues and policy directions.* International journal of humanities and social science, 2011. **1**(21): p. 205-223.

[140] Wegener, H.C., *Antibiotics in animal feed and their role in resistance development.* Current opinion in microbiology, 2003. **6**(5): p. 439-445.

[141] Barton, M.D., *Antibiotic use in animal feed and its impact on human health.* Nutrition research reviews, 2000. **13**(2): p. 279-299.

[142] Franklin, A.M., et al., *Antibiotics in agroecosystems: introduction to the special section.* Journal of environmental quality, 2016. **45**(2): p. 377-393.

[143] Iwu, C.D., L. Korsten, and A.I. Okoh, *The incidence of antibiotic resistance within and beyond the agricultural ecosystem: A concern for public health.* MicrobiologyOpen, 2020: p. e1035.

[144] Manyi-Loh, C., et al., *Antibiotic Use in Agriculture and Its Consequential Resistance in Environmental Sources: Potential Public Health Implications.* Molecules (Basel, Switzerland), 2018. **23**(4): p. 795.

[145] Laxminarayan, R., et al., *Antibiotic resistance—the need for global solutions.* The Lancet infectious diseases, 2013. **13**(12): p. 1057-1098.

[146] Finch, R. and P. Hunter, *Antibiotic resistance—action to promote new technologies: report of an EU Intergovernmental Conference held in Birmingham, UK, 12-13 December 2005.* Journal of Antimicrobial Chemotherapy, 2006. **58**(suppl_1): p. i3-i22.

[147] Szekeres, E., et al., *Investigating antibiotics, antibiotic resistance genes, and microbial contaminants in groundwater in relation to the proximity of urban areas.* Environmental Pollution, 2018. **236**: p. 734-744.

[148] Segura, P.A., et al., *Review of the occurrence of anti-infectives in contaminated wastewaters and natural and drinking waters.* Environmental health perspectives, 2009. **117**(5): p. 675-684.

[149] MacFadden, D.R., et al., *Antibiotic resistance increases with local temperature.*

Nature Climate Change, 2018. **8**(6): p. 510-514.

[150] Blair, J.M., *A climate for antibiotic resistance.* Nature Climate Change, 2018. **8**(6): p. 460-461.

[151] Akhtar, A.Z., et al., *Health professionals' roles in animal agriculture, climate change, and human health.* American journal of preventive medicine, 2009. **36**(2): p. 182-187.

[152] Springmann, M., et al., *Global and regional health effects of future food production under climate change: a modelling study.* Lancet, 2016. **387**(10031): p. 1937-46.

[153] Despommier, D., *The vertical farm: feeding the world in the 21st century.* 2010: Macmillan.

[154] Hill, M.K., *Understanding environmental pollution.* 2020: Cambridge University Press.

[155] Ahmed, N., S. Thompson, and M. Glaser, *Global aquaculture productivity, environmental sustainability, and climate change adaptability.* Environmental management, 2019. **63**(2): p. 159-172.

[156] Clements, J.C. and T. Chopin, *Ocean acidification and marine aquaculture in North America: potential impacts and mitigation strategies.* Reviews in Aquaculture, 2017. **9**(4): p. 326-341.

[157] Phlips, E.J., et al., *Hurricanes, El Niño and harmful algal blooms in two sub-tropical Florida estuaries: Direct and indirect impacts.* Scientific reports, 2020. **10**(1): p. 1-12.

[158] Kundzewicz, Z.W., et al., *Flood risk and climate change: global and regional perspectives.* Hydrological Sciences Journal, 2014. **59**(1): p. 1-28.

[159] Van Aalst, M.K., *The impacts of climate change on the risk of natural disasters.* Disasters, 2006. **30**(1): p. 5-18.

[160] Agrawala, S., et al., *Development and climate change in Bangladesh: focus on coastal flooding and the Sundarbans.* 2003: Citeseer.

[161] Brammer, H., *Bangladesh's dynamic coastal regions and sea-level rise.* Climate Risk Management, 2014. **1**: p. 51-62.

[162] Thanvisitthpon, N., S. Shrestha, and I. Pal, *Urban flooding and climate change: a case study of Bangkok, Thailand.* Environment and Urbanization ASIA, 2018. **9**(1): p. 86-100.

[163] Carbognin, L., et al., *Global change and relative sea level rise at Venice: what impact in term of flooding.* Climate Dynamics, 2010. **35**(6): p. 1039-1047.

[164] Wdowinski, S., et al., *Increasing flooding hazard in coastal communities due to rising sea level: Case study of Miami Beach, Florida.* Ocean & Coastal Management, 2016. **126**: p. 1-8.

[165] Zaalberg, R., et al., *Prevention, adaptation, and threat denial: Flooding experiences in the Netherlands.* Risk Analysis: An International Journal, 2009. **29**(12): p. 1759-1778.

[166] McCann, D.G., A. Moore, and M.-E. Walker, *The water/health nexus in disaster medicine: I. Drought versus flood.* Current Opinion in Environmental Sustainability, 2011. **3**(6): p. 480-485.

[167] Sivakumar, M.V., *Impacts of natural disasters in agriculture: An overview.* World Meteorological Organisation, Geneva, Switzerland, 2014.

[168] Marchigiani, R., et al., *Wind disasters: A comprehensive review of current management strategies.* International journal of critical illness and injury science, 2013. **3**(2): p. 130.

[169] Hunter, P.R., *Climate change and waterborne and vector-borne disease.* Journal of applied microbiology, 2003. **94**: p. 37-46.

[170] Davies, G.I., et al., *Water-borne diseases and extreme weather events in Cambodia: Review of impacts and implications of climate change.* International journal of environmental research and public health, 2015. **12**(1): p. 191-213.

[171] White, I., *Water and the city: Risk, resilience and planning for a sustainable future*. 2013: Routledge.

[172] Price-Smith, A.T., *The health of nations: infectious disease, environmental change, and their effects on national security and development*. 2001: Mit Press.

[173] Rahman, S.U., *Impacts of flood on the lives and livelihoods of people in Bangladesh: A case study of a village in Manikganj district*. 2014, BRAC University.

[174] Ramachandra, T. and P.P. Mujumdar, *Urban floods: Case study of Bangalore.* Disaster Dev, 2009. **3**(2): p. 1-98.

[175] Levy, K., et al., *Untangling the impacts of climate change on waterborne diseases: a systematic review of relationships between diarrheal diseases and temperature, rainfall, flooding, and drought.* Environmental science & technology, 2016. **50**(10): p. 4905-4922.

[176] Ten Veldhuis, J., et al., *Microbial risks associated with exposure to pathogens in contaminated urban flood water.* Water research, 2010. **44**(9): p. 2910-2918.

[177] Nasci, R.S. and C.G. Moore, *Vector-borne disease surveillance and natural disasters.* Emerging Infectious Diseases, 1998. **4**(2): p. 333.

[178] Anyamba, A., et al., *Prediction, assessment of the Rift Valley fever activity in East and Southern Africa 2006-2008 and possible vector control strategies.* The American journal of tropical medicine

and hygiene, 2010. **83**(2_Suppl): p. 43-51.

[179] Kouadio, I.K., et al., *Infectious diseases following natural disasters: prevention and control measures.* Expert review of anti-infective therapy, 2012. **10**(1): p. 95-104.

[180] Adeloye, A.J. and R. Rustum, *Lagos (Nigeria) flooding and influence of urban planning.* Proceedings of the Institution of Civil Engineers-Urban Design and Planning, 2011. **164**(3): p. 175-187.

[181] Landesman, L.Y., *Public health management of disasters: the practice guide.* 2005: American public health association.

[182] Cash, R.A., et al., *Reducing the health effect of natural hazards in Bangladesh.* The Lancet, 2013. **382**(9910): p. 2094-2103.

[183] Chan, N.W., *Impacts of disasters and disaster risk management in Malaysia: The case of floods*, in *Resilience and recovery in Asian disasters*. 2015, Springer. p. 239-265.

[184] Pelling, M., et al., *Reducing disaster risk: a challenge for development*. 2004.

[185] Le, N.K., et al., *International Health Security: A Summative Assessment by ACAIM Consensus Group*, in *Contemporary Developments and Perspectives in International Health Security - Volume 1*. 2020, IntechOpen: London, UK. p. 1-34.

[186] O'Neill, M.S. and K.L. Ebi, *Temperature extremes and health: impacts of climate variability and change in the United States.* Journal of Occupational and Environmental Medicine, 2009. **51**(1): p. 13-25.

[187] Marsa, L., *Fevered: Why a Hotter Planet Will Hurt Our Health-and How We Can Save Ourselves*. 2013: Rodale.

[188] Reddy, P.P., *Impacts of climate change on agriculture*, in *Climate resilient agriculture for ensuring food security*. 2015, Springer. p. 43-90.

[189] Lippsett, L. and G. Warming, *Storms, Floods, and Droughts*. Oceanus, 2012. **49**(3): p. 20.

[190] Goudie, A.S., *Dust storms: Recent developments*. Journal of environmental management, 2009. **90**(1): p. 89-94.

[191] Peng, W., et al., *A review of historical and recent locust outbreaks: Links to global warming, food security and mitigation strategies*. Environmental Research, 2020. **191**: p. 110046.

[192] Nadal-Sala, D., et al., *Global warming likely to enhance black locust (Robinia pseudoacacia L.) growth in a Mediterranean riparian forest*. Forest Ecology and Management, 2019. **449**: p. 117448.

[193] Salih, A.A., et al., *Climate change and locust outbreak in East Africa*. Nature Climate Change, 2020. **10**(7): p. 584-585.

[194] Sun, Q., et al., *Global heat stress on health, wildfires, and agricultural crops under different levels of climate warming*. Environment international, 2019. **128**: p. 125-136.

[195] Rappold, A.G., et al., *Forecast-based interventions can reduce the health and economic burden of wildfires*. Environmental science & technology, 2014. **48**(18): p. 10571-10579.

[196] Della-Marta, P.M., et al., *Doubled length of western European summer heat waves since 1880*. Journal of Geophysical Research: Atmospheres, 2007. **112**(D15).

[197] Kent, S.T., et al., *Heat waves and health outcomes in Alabama (USA): the importance of heat wave definition*. Environmental health perspectives, 2014. **122**(2): p. 151-158.

[198] Smith, T.T., B.F. Zaitchik, and J.M. Gohlke, *Heat waves in the United States: definitions, patterns and trends*. Climatic change, 2013. **118**(3-4): p. 811-825.

[199] Anderson, G.B. and M.L. Bell, *Heat waves in the United States: mortality risk during heat waves and effect modification by heat wave characteristics in 43 US communities*. Environmental health perspectives, 2011. **119**(2): p. 210-218.

[200] Fouillet, A., et al., *Excess mortality related to the August 2003 heat wave in France*. International archives of occupational and environmental health, 2006. **80**(1): p. 16-24.

[201] Johnson, H., et al., *The impact of the 2003 heat wave on daily mortality in England and Wales and the use of rapid weekly mortality estimates*. Euro surveillance: bulletin européen sur les maladies transmissibles= European communicable disease bulletin, 2005. **10**(7): p. 168-171.

[202] Stawicki, S.P., et al., *Comorbidity polypharmacy score and its clinical utility: A pragmatic practitioner's perspective*. Journal of emergencies, trauma, and shock, 2015. **8**(4): p. 224.

[203] Mubang, R.N., et al., *Comorbidity– Polypharmacy Score as predictor of outcomes in older trauma patients: a retrospective validation study*. World journal of surgery, 2015. **39**(8): p. 2068-2075.

[204] Tolentino, J.C., et al., *Comorbidity-polypharmacy score predicts readmissions and in-hospital mortality: A six-hospital health network experience*. Journal of Basic and Clinical Pharmacy, 2017. **8**(3).

[205] Cohen, M.S., et al., *Patient frailty: Key considerations, definitions, and practical implications*. Challenges in Elder Care, 2016: p. 9.

[206] Keatinge, W.R., et al., *Increased platelet and red cell counts, blood viscosity,*

and plasma cholesterol levels during heat stress, and mortality from coronary and cerebral thrombosis. The American journal of medicine, 1986. **81**(5): p. 795-800.

[207] Kenny, G.P., et al., *Heat stress in older individuals and patients with common chronic diseases.* Cmaj, 2010. **182**(10): p. 1053-1060.

[208] Szema, A.M., *Asthma, hay fever, pollen, and climate change*, in *Global Climate Change and Public Health.* 2014, Springer. p. 155-165.

[209] Smith, J.B. and D.A. Tirpak, *The potential effects of global climate change on the United States: Report to Congress.* Vol. 1. 1989: US Environmental Protection Agency, Office of Policy, Planning, and ....

[210] Kunzli, N., et al., *Health effects of the 2003 Southern California wildfires on children.* American journal of respiratory and critical care medicine, 2006. **174**(11): p. 1221-1228.

[211] Friedli, H., et al., *Volatile organic trace gases emitted from North American wildfires.* Global biogeochemical cycles, 2001. **15**(2): p. 435-452.

[212] Easterling, D.R., *Recent changes in frost days and the frost-free season in the United States.* Bulletin of the American Meteorological Society, 2002. **83**(9): p. 1327-1332.

[213] Matyasovszky, I., et al., *Biogeographical drivers of ragweed pollen concentrations in Europe.* Theoretical and Applied Climatology, 2018. **133**(1-2): p. 277-295.

[214] Dougherty, R. and J.V. Fahy, *Acute exacerbations of asthma: epidemiology, biology and the exacerbation-prone phenotype.* Clinical & Experimental Allergy, 2009. **39**(2): p. 193-202.

[215] Forman, R.T., *Urban ecology: science of cities.* 2014: Cambridge University Press.

[216] Doerr, S.H. and C. Santín, *Global trends in wildfire and its impacts: perceptions versus realities in a changing world.* Philosophical transactions of the Royal Society of London. Series B, Biological sciences, 2016. **371**(1696): p. 20150345.

[217] Kelly, F.J. and J.C. Fussell, *Global nature of airborne particle toxicity and health effects: a focus on megacities, wildfires, dust storms and residential biomass burning.* Toxicology Research, 2020. **9**(4): p. 331-345.

[218] Ghasemizadeh, R. and H. Taheri, *Monitoring dust storms in drylands using GIS (Case study: Dust storm in Iran, July 2009).* 2009.

[219] Bari, M.A. and W.B. Kindzierski, *Fine particulate matter (PM2. 5) in Edmonton, Canada: Source apportionment and potential risk for human health.* Environmental Pollution, 2016. **218**: p. 219-229.

[220] Teather, K., et al., *Examining the links between air quality, climate change and respiratory health in Qatar.* Avicenna, 2013. **2013**(1): p. 9.

[221] Wettstein, Z.S., et al., *Cardiovascular and cerebrovascular emergency department visits associated with wildfire smoke exposure in California in 2015.* Journal of the American heart association, 2018. 7(8): p. e007492.

[222] Liu, J.C. and R.D. Peng, *The impact of wildfire smoke on compositions of fine particulate matter by ecoregion in the Western US.* Journal of Exposure Science & Environmental Epidemiology, 2019. **29**(6): p. 765-776.

[223] Nordhaus, W.D., *The economics of hurricanes and implications of global warming.* Climate Change Economics, 2010. **1**(01): p. 1-20.

[224] Tamura, Y. and S. Cao, *International group for wind-related disaster risk*

reduction (IG-WRDRR). Journal of wind engineering and industrial aerodynamics, 2012. **104**: p. 3-11.

[225] Pielke Jr, R.A., et al., *Hurricanes and global warming.* Bulletin of the American Meteorological Society, 2005. **86**(11): p. 1571-1576.

[226] González-Alemán, J.J., et al., *Potential increase in hazard from Mediterranean hurricane activity with global warming.* Geophysical Research Letters, 2019. **46**(3): p. 1754-1764.

[227] Chen, X. *Relationship Between Global Warming and Hurricanes Wind Speed Based on Analyzing MODIS Remote Sensing Data.* in *Proceedings of the Sixth International Forum on Decision Sciences.* 2020. Springer.

[228] Siegel, V., W.E. Rich, and M. Mahany, *2020 hurricane season during COVID-19.* 2020.

[229] Filipe, J.F., et al., *Floods, Hurricanes, and Other Catastrophes: A Challenge for the Immune System of Livestock and Other Animals.* Frontiers in Veterinary Science, 2020. **7**: p. 16.

[230] Welch-Devine, M. and B. Orland, *Is It Time to Move Away? How Hurricanes Affect Future Plans.* International Journal of Mass Emergencies & Disasters, 2020. **38**(1).

[231] Lenane, Z., et al., *Association of post-traumatic stress disorder symptoms following Hurricane Katrina with incident cardiovascular disease events among older adults with hypertension.* The American Journal of Geriatric Psychiatry, 2019. **27**(3): p. 310-321.

[232] Espinel, Z., et al., *Climate-driven Atlantic hurricanes pose rising threats for psychopathology.* The Lancet Psychiatry, 2019. **6**(9): p. 721-723.

[233] Honoré, R.L., *Speaking Truth to Power on How Hurricane Katrina Beat Us.* 2020, American Public Health Association.

[234] Becquart, N.A., et al., *Cardiovascular disease hospitalizations in Louisiana parishes' elderly before, during and after hurricane Katrina.* International journal of environmental research and public health, 2019. **16**(1): p. 74.

[235] Raker, E.J., et al., *Twelve years later: The long-term mental health consequences of Hurricane Katrina.* Social Science & Medicine, 2019. **242**: p. 112610.

[236] Cohen, G.H., et al., *Improved social services and the burden of post-traumatic stress disorder among economically vulnerable people after a natural disaster: a modelling study.* The Lancet Planetary Health, 2019. **3**(2): p. e93-e101.

[237] Swim, J., et al., *Psychology and global climate change: Addressing a multi-faceted phenomenon and set of challenges. A report by the American Psychological Association's task force on the interface between psychology and global climate change.* American Psychological Association, Washington, 2009.

[238] Beyerl, K., H.A. Mieg, and E. Weber, *Comparing perceived effects of climate-related environmental change and adaptation strategies for the Pacific small island states of Tuvalu, Samoa, and Tonga.* Island Studies Journal, 2018. **13**(1): p. 25-44.

[239] Raleigh, C. and H. Urdal, *Climate change, environmental degradation and armed conflict.* Political geography, 2007. **26**(6): p. 674-694.

[240] Scheffran, J. and A. Battaglini, *Climate and conflicts: the security risks of global warming.* Regional Environmental Change, 2011. **11**(1): p. 27-39.

[241] Abel, G.J., et al., *Climate, conflict and forced migration.* Global Environmental Change, 2019. **54**: p. 239-249.

[242] Gallant, K., *The Nexus of Climate, Crops, and Conflict in the Horn of Africa*. 2020.

[243] Shultz, J.M., et al., *Public health and mental health implications of environmentally induced forced migration*. Disaster medicine and public health preparedness, 2019. **13**(2): p. 116-122.

[244] Trombley, J., S. Chalupka, and L. Anderko, *Climate change and mental health*. AJN The American Journal of Nursing, 2017. **117**(4): p. 44-52.

[245] Grace, D., *Food Safety in Low and Middle Income Countries*. Int J Environ Res Public Health, 2015. **12**(9): p. 10490-507.

[246] Purgato, M., et al., *Psychological therapies for the treatment of mental disorders in low- and middle-income countries affected by humanitarian crises*. Cochrane Database Syst Rev, 2018. 7: p. CD011849.

[247] Oliver-Smith, A., *Climate change and population displacement: disasters and diasporas in the twenty-first century*. Anthropology and climate change. From encounters to actions, 2009: p. 116-136.

[248] Weir, T. and Z. Virani, *Three linked risks for development in the Pacific Islands: climate change, disasters and conflict*. Climate and Development, 2011. **3**(3): p. 193-208.

[249] McMichael, C., J. Barnett, and A.J. McMichael, *An ill wind? Climate change, migration, and health*. Environmental health perspectives, 2012. **120**(5): p. 646-654.

[250] Hoegh-Guldberg, O., et al., *Impacts of 1.5 C global warming on natural and human systems*. Global warming of 1.5° C. An IPCC Special Report, 2018.

[251] McCarthy, M.P., M.J. Best, and R.A. Betts, *Climate change in cities due to global warming and urban effects*.

Geophysical research letters, 2010. **37**(9).

[252] Athanasiou, T., *Divided planet: The ecology of rich and poor*. 1998: University of Georgia Press.

[253] Tsavoussis, A., et al., *Child-witnessed domestic violence and its adverse effects on brain development: a call for societal self-examination and awareness*. Frontiers in public health, 2014. 2: p. 178.

[254] Tsavoussis, A., S.P. Stawicki, and T.J. Papadimos, *Child-witnessed domestic violence: An epidemic in the shadows*. International journal of critical illness and injury science, 2015. **5**(1): p. 64.

[255] Paladino, L., et al., *Reflections on the Ebola public health emergency of international concern, part 2: the unseen epidemic of posttraumatic stress among health-care personnel and survivors of the 2014-2016 Ebola outbreak*. Journal of Global Infectious Diseases, 2017. **9**(2): p. 45.

[256] O'Neill, S., et al., *Patterns of suicidal ideation and behavior in Northern Ireland and associations with conflict related trauma*. PLoS One, 2014. **9**(3): p. e91532.

[257] Butryn, T., et al., *The shortage of psychiatrists and other mental health providers: causes, current state, and potential solutions*. International Journal of Academic Medicine, 2017. **3**(1): p. 5.

[258] Bruckner, T.A., et al., *The mental health workforce gap in low-and middle-income countries: a needs-based approach*. Bulletin of the World Health Organization, 2011. **89**: p. 184-194.

[259] Burns, J.K., *Mental health services funding and development in KwaZulu-Natal: a tale of inequity and neglect*. South African Medical Journal, 2010. **100**(10): p. 662-666.

[260] Morris, J., et al., *Global mental health resources and services: a WHO survey of 184 countries.* Public Health Reviews, 2012. **34**(2): p. 1-19.

[261] Padhy, S.K., et al., *Mental health effects of climate change.* Indian journal of occupational and environmental medicine, 2015. **19**(1): p. 3.

[262] Fritze, J.G., et al., *Hope, despair and transformation: climate change and the promotion of mental health and wellbeing.* International journal of mental health systems, 2008. **2**(1): p. 1-10.

[263] Glanz, K., B.K. Rimer, and K. Viswanath, *Health behavior and health education: theory, research, and practice.* 2008: John Wiley & Sons.

[264] Hahn, R.A. and B.I. Truman, *Education improves public health and promotes health equity.* International journal of health services, 2015. **45**(4): p. 657-678.

[265] Fazel, M., et al., *Mental health interventions in schools in high-income countries.* The Lancet Psychiatry, 2014. **1**(5): p. 377-387.

[266] Parker, C.L., *Slowing global warming: benefits for patients and the planet.* American family physician, 2011. **84**(3): p. 271-278.

Chapter 10

The Social and Health Impact of Accidents at Work: The Analysis of the Italian Case

Romano Benini

Abstract

The months of a gradual exit from the pandemic show some significant data and phenomena regarding the phenomenon of accidents at work and occupational diseases. The Italian figure highlights a recovery in injuries and illnesses, but also in the impact of new risk factors deriving from the digitalization of work, which grew with smart working during the pandemic. At the same time, the new organizational models highlight the increased risk of work-related stress diseases. The Italian situation makes clear the need to intervene on the issue of organizational well-being and welfare, to limit the negative impact of risk factors associated with this economic system on society and the health system through a new work culture.

Keywords: accidents at work, inclusion, welfare, risk prevention, work-related stress

1. Introduction

Italy is the second country in Europe for manufacturing production and the nation week in the world from the point of view of industrialization, albeit with a limited territory and population. For many decades, this process of industrialization has had to face various problems relating to situations of risk of accidents at work. Each economic phase involves the definition of different risk conditions. The passage from the industrial model to a tertiary economy and to the "Fourth capitalism" has led many countries to the overcoming of the central function of manufacturing production, for the promotion of a system based on services. This has also happened to countries with a great industrial tradition, such as Italy and Germany. However, this situation has not entirely limited the conditions of exposure to the risk of accidents at work: the maintenance of a significant presence in industrial production has been accompanied by the new risk conditions that characterize the new economic models and which extend to the sector of tertiary and services. For this reason, in the last 20 years, Italian legislation and the system of employment contracts have placed a strong focus on the prevention of risks at work, introducing important obligations for each company and specific figures, such as the Safety Manager. Italy has a very significant law regarding the prevention and protection of health and safety in the workplace, the "Consolidated text for health and safety in the workplace" [1] (Legislative Decree no. 81 of 2008), a national body called Inail which carries out insurance activities, but also for the prevention of occupational risks, information, training, and assistance in the field of safety and health at work and a national inspection agency for checks in companies. However, the issue of exposure to the risk of accidents at work remains a very present phenomenon, which must be considered due to the following in-depth elements, which constitute important aspects of the evolution of the economic and production system, destined to produce effects also in the coming years:

- The presence of conditions of exposure to the risk of accidents in small industrial enterprises, in subcontracting and in less structured production contexts;

- The evolution of risk characteristics due to technological innovation and digitalization and in the tertiary and service sectors;

- The presence, in addition to the risk of accidents and injuries, of increasing exposure to pathologies connected to the phenomenon of "work-related stress".

This situation must be seen as a whole and determines significant impacts on society and on the health of citizens, which is useful to examine and evaluate.

2. The methodology used for the analysis of the reference data

The primary source of the analysis contained in this essay is the Information System of accidents reported to Inail, the Italian public institution that has insurance and preventive functions to combat the phenomenon of accidents at work. This database is extremely detailed and updated every 3 months and in particular evaluates the trends in the different types of accidents and for the different territories. However, the hypothetical assessment of unreported accidents, especially present in some economic areas and territories, was also taken into consideration. The focus on work-related stress takes into account the compensation claims submitted by workers to Inail, but also in this case the trend phenomenon is taken into account, as many situations may not have been reported. The methodology, therefore, considers the empirical and factual datum, but completes this datum through a phenomenological evaluation of the current trends, in the face of the possibility of having a complaint that does not correspond to all situations of injury or risk. In particular, with respect to the impact of digitization and the role of smart work, a survey carried out by the Foundation for Labor Consultants was considered on a statistically significant sample.

This essay, therefore, proposes, as an innovation of the methodology for the analysis of the evolution of the risk of accidents at work and the worsening of safety conditions, the evaluation, and consideration of factual data deriving from official reports of accidents, including reports of work-related stress, to the public institution Inail, in connection with the phenomenological analysis of trends, supported by correct surveys on an evaluation level. In this way, a more complete assessment of the reality and extent of the phenomena and the evolution of risk factors can be connected to the analysis of what has actually been reported.

Among the various initiatives of Istat, the Italian national research body for statistics, aimed at gathering the information necessary for the analysis of the effects of the health crisis on the economy and society, in May and November 2020, two specific surveys aimed at understanding how Italian companies have experienced such a dramatic phase, with particular reference to the economic, financial and employment impact. These researches constitute an important component in defining the proposed methodological framework.

3. The current situation and 2020 data

The phenomenon of accidents at work in Italy is read through the data of the complaints to Inail and shows how the first months of economic recovery in 2021 led to an increase in risk situations and accidents. Among other things, it must be taken into account how reporting to Inail represents a legal and correct method of verifying the accident phenomenon, but how in Italy there is the problem of accidents not reported to the national insurance institution, especially in situations concerning the conditions of irregular work, present above all in some sectors. In any case, the latest Inail report of 2021 [2] shows an increase in the accident phenomenon of particular significance. In the period January–August of this year, compared to the same period of 2020, there was an increase in overall accident reports, a decrease in fatal ones, and a rise in occupational diseases. The reports of accidents at work submitted to Inail by last August [3] were 349,449, over 27,000 more (+ 8.5%) compared to 322,132 in the first 8 months of 2020, a summary of a decrease in complaints observed in the quarter. January–March (−11%) and an increase in the April–August period (+ 26%) in the comparison between the 2 years. The data collected on 31 August of each year show in the first 8 months of 2021 a national increase in accidents while commuting, that is, those occurring on the return journey between the home and the workplace (+ 20.6%, from 38,001 to 45,821 cases), which decreased by 32% in the first 2 months of this year and increased by 59% in the period March–August (thanks to the massive use of smart working last year, starting from March), and an increase of 6.9% (from 284,131 to 303,628) in those occurred on the occasion of work, which fell by 10% in the first quarter of this year and increased by 22% in the April–August period. The number of reported work accidents increased by 6.9% in the Industry and Services insurance management, by 3.6% in Agriculture, and by 29.2% in the state sector. The territorial analysis shows a decrease in complaints only in the North-West (−3.6%), as opposed to the Islands (+ 16.5%), the South (+ 14.9%), the Center (+14, 5%), and the North-East (+ 13.6%).

The increase that emerges from the comparison of the first 8 months of 2020 and 2021 [4] is linked only to the male component, which records a + 14.7% (from 195,612 to 224,400 complaints), while the female one is down by 1.2% (from 126,520 to 125,049). The increase affected both Italian workers (+ 7.8%) and non-EU (+ 14.5%) and EU workers (+ 2.5%). The analysis by age group shows a decline only among the 15–19 year olds (−0.7%), with increases for the 20–49 year-old group (+ 9.9%) and among the over 50s (+3, 5%).

The reports of accidents at work with a fatal outcome submitted to the Institute by August were 772, 51 less than the 823 recorded in the first 8 months of 2020 (−6.2%). The comparison between 2020 and 2021 requires caution as the data of the fatal reports of the monthly open data, more than those of the reports as a whole, are provisional and strongly influenced by the covid-19 pandemic, with the result of not counting a significant number of "late" fatal reports of contagion, in particular relating to the month of March 2020. At the national level, the data collected on 31 August of each year show an increase only in cases occurring in progress for the first 8 months of this year, went from 138 to 152 (+ 10.1%), while those at work were 65 less (from 685 to 620, −9.5%). The decrease observed in the comparison between the first 8 months of 2020 and 2021 is linked both to the female component, whose fatal cases reported went from 83 to 78 (−6.0%) and to the male component, which went from 740 to 694 cases (−6.2%). The decrease concerns the complaints of Italian workers (from 700 to 663) and EU workers (from 41 to 25), while those of non-EU workers went from 82 to 84.

As of August 31, 2021, 12 multiple accidents occurred in the first 8 months for a total of 29 deaths, 17 of which were road accidents. Last year, however, there were six multiple accidents recorded between January and August, with 12 fatal cases reported, half of which were road accidents. The complaints of occupational disease registered by Inail in the first 8 months of 2021 were 36,496, 8735 more than in the same period of 2020 (+ 31.5%), a summary of a decrease of 26% in the January–February period and of an increase of 66% in that of March–August, in the comparison between the 2 years.

The pathologies reported, therefore, start to increase again, after 2020 strongly conditioned by the pandemic with reports in a constant decrease in comparison with previous years [5–7]. In fact, last year, arrests and restarts of production activities reduced exposure to the risk of contracting occupational diseases. Pathologies of the osteo-muscular system and connective tissue, of the nervous system, and of the ear continue to represent, even in the first months of 2021, the first three occupational diseases reported, followed by tumors, which exceed those of the respiratory system in August.

This situation, which exposes the data of the national information system of Inail, provides for interventions on the system of rules, which the Italian government has announced and which also concern the strengthening of inspection and control activities. However, it seems important to point out the impact that the accident phenomenon continues to have on the social and health system and how the evolution of the economic system has introduced some risk factors that can be addressed not only through increased controls but also through different ways of carrying out the work performance, greater attention to organizational well-being and a widespread introduction of corporate welfare tools. The accident data does not derive only from the introduction of dangerous work tools and the lack of controls in some sectors, but is often a consequence of excessive workloads, the acceleration of work times, and a "culture of performance" and productivity which increases risk margins and which, when it does not cause an injury, in any case, causes an increase in the condition of "work-related stress" [8–10].

4. The phenomenon of accidents for working women

In this context, it becomes useful to analyze the impact of the phenomenon of accidents on the female component of Italian work. Also in this case it becomes useful to analyze the trends shown by the Inail database on the evolution of accident reports reported is more present. This makes this assessment partly underestimated. However, the data show us that in some situations it is women who appear to be more exposed to greater conditions of risk. If we analyze the most consolidated annual Inail data in the period between 2015 and 2019, accident reports [11–13] presented to Inail increased overall by 1.3% (from 636,674 in 2015 to 644,970 in 2019).

Faced with an increase in female employment equal to +1.1% 1, the complaints and accidents of female workers went from 227,068 in 2015 to 231,128 in 2019, equal to a percentage increase of 1.8%, higher than that recorded among male workers (+ 1.0%), for which Istat recorded an increase in employment equal to +0.3%. In the same 5 year period, the incidence of women in total accidents was almost constant and on average equal to 35.8%. On the other hand, reports of accidents with fatal outcomes among female workers decreased, from 117 cases in 2015 to 97 in 2019, equal to −17.1%, more markedly than the 8.9% reduction recorded over the same period of time among workers. It is important to point out that the incidence of accidents for female workers is particularly high in the domestic and family services sector (domestic workers and carers), with 89.9%

of the total complaints in the sector, followed by health and social assistance (74, 2%) and from the packaging of clothing items (70.9%), while in the riskiest sectors of the industry it drops to 2.8% recorded in construction. The complaints related to the insurance policy against domestic accidents (mandatory for all people aged between 18 and 67 who take care of the home in a habitual, exclusive, and free-way), in 2019 were a total of 760 and registered an exceptional increase of 58.3% compared to 2018, when 480 were registered. Almost all (742) concerned women and no cases with a fatal outcome were recorded in 2019, compared to 20 cases in 2015–2018. A truly significant figure is that which concerns the overall complaints of accidents at work "in progress", that is, occurring on the return journey between home and work, which continue to be for female workers, even in 2019, more than men: 54,299 cases against 51,524. In relative terms, ongoing cases represent 23.5% (practically one in four) of female complaints (231.128) and 12.5% (just over one in ten) of male ones (413.779). For complaints with a fatal outcome, the incidence of this type of accident among female workers is even higher: in 2019, almost one in two female deaths (44 out of 97, 45.4%) occurred in progress, a ratio that for men dropped to about one in four (281 out of 1087, 25.9%). A gender difference that is confirmed by looking at the broader category of accidents "outside the company" (sum of all accidents while traveling and those during work occurring with the means of transport involved) generally attributable to the risk of road traffic: 25.3% (58,396) of female complaints against 16.1% (66,485) of male ones.

5. Data analysis

For a correct analysis of the phenomenon of accidents, it is necessary to consider how, in addition to issues of a cultural nature, one of the major problems concerning the scourge of deaths and accidents at work—in Italy and beyond—is that relating to the measurement of the phenomenon as when comparing the data between countries, the incidence rates are difficult to interpret. In fact, the probability of going into an injury is, among other factors, related to the work activity that the worker carries out and the weight of the different economic activities varies from one country to another depending on the structure of each economy. Furthermore, a higher number of accidents ascertained at work does not necessarily indicate worse safety conditions; on the contrary, it may indicate a greater propensity to report and therefore paradoxically better protection of the worker. It should also be considered that among the various injured, sick, and dead at work, there is a part of workers in irregular conditions that are difficult to estimate. It should also be considered how in Europe those accidents on the way from home to work or vice versa are not considered in the data, i.e., accidents "in itinere", which the Italian system instead evaluates and considers from an insurance point of view. In any case, if we consider the pre-Covid data, Italy ranks above the EU28 average (1.8) for the number of deaths at work out of the total number of employees, with 2.3 deaths per 100,000 employed. Among the states most similar to Italy, France recorded a higher figure (2.7); the United Kingdom (0.8), Germany (0.8), and Spain (2) a lower figure. The phenomenon of unreported accidents should also be considered: the "Independent Observatory of Bologna on the fallen from work" believes that a high number of deaths at work escapes the statistics on the phenomenon [14]. This observatory includes in its data irregular workers, unreported deaths, and a portion of fatal injuries not ascertained by Inail. According to the independent Bolognese Observatory, 2019 would even have ended with 1437 workers who died at work: 701 in the workplace, 736 in transit; a figure double that of Inail.

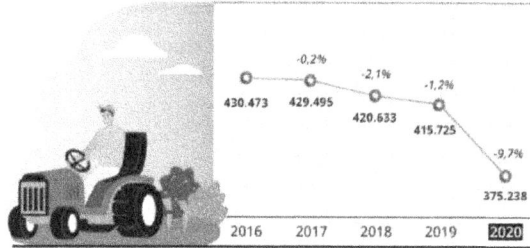

Figure 1.
Variation in accidents.

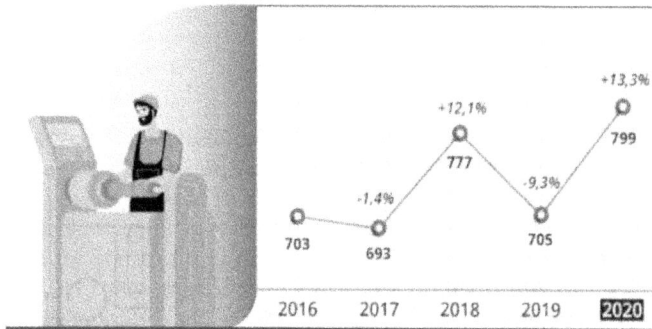

Figure 2.
Variation in fatal cases.

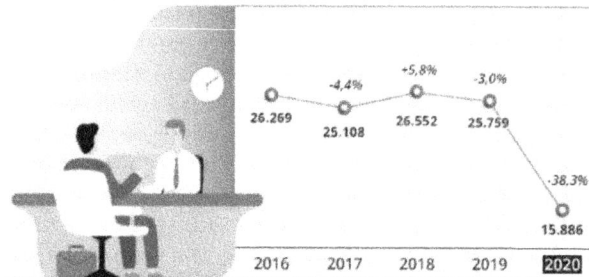

Figure 3.
Variation in occupational diseases.

In any case, the accident phenomenon represents a very present reality for Italy and with the increase in accidents coinciding with the resumption of post-Covid economic activities, it appears important to initiate careful preventive action, which also concerns the culture of health at work itself. In this effort, it is also important to point out how risk factors are often linked to the rhythms imposed on the job and not only to a lack of attention to prevention. The data on the evolution of work-related stress and related pathologies constitutes an interesting aspect in this sense (**Figures 1–3**).

6. The advanced tertiary sector and related work stress

If construction and manufacturing activities are still the most significant components of the accident phenomenon, the issue of occupational diseases, with their relative impact on the health system, increasingly concerns the tertiary sector as well. In this context, the phenomenon of work-related stress has grown in recent years, linked to increasingly widespread pathologies. Work-related stress occurs among workers when the demands made on them exceed the ability to cope with it, with harmful consequences for health and mental balance, which are also reflected in the relational life of those affected. Some examples of working conditions that involve psychosocial risks and which could therefore cause work-related stress are:

- Excessive workloads;

- Conflicting requests or lack of clarity on roles;

- Lack of involvement in decision-making processes affecting workers;

- Inadequate management of organizational changes, job insecurity;

- Ineffective communication, lack of support from colleagues or superiors;

- Physical and psychological violence against the worker, perpetrated by the employer or by third parties.

- From these situations, characterized by a strong dysfunctional protracted over time, symptoms may arise that can cause real occupational diseases:

- Psycho-emotional such as anxiety, fear, obsession, hypochondria, hysteria, paranoia, depression, aggression, low self-esteem, and sleep disturbances, which amplify the risk factors for neuropsychiatric diseases;

- Physical, affecting organs and systems such as the cardiovascular system (with consequent arterial hypertension), the gastrointestinal system (with gastritis, gastric ulcer, and ulcerative colitis), the osteoarticular system (with pain in the spine, scapulohumeral periarthritis, and muscle tension), or immune or psycho-somatic pathologies (such as dermatitis, psoriasis, hyperhidrosis, skin rashes);

- Behavioral, which amplify the risks of accidents, alcoholism, smoking, drug addiction and also compromise the relational and family balance of the worker.

Intense and prolonged stress over time can cause psychosomatic, physical, mental, and behavioral disorders, even severe ones, in workers, with more or less stable effects.

By analyzing the relationship between work-related stress and some pathologies, in fact, a directly proportional correlation was identified between the risk of psychological deficit and an increase in work stress. The conditions most often encountered range from mood disorders, to alterations in the sleep-wake rhythm, to interpersonal and family conflicts, up to burnout and depression. A pre-existing psychophysical disorder, such as that of adaptation or post-traumatic stress disorder, can also coexist with one related to work events, sometimes strengthening it. Alongside these psychosomatic and behavioral disorders, the consequences of prolonged work-related stress can also affect the cardiovascular and nervous, endocrine, gastrointestinal, and immune systems. There is also a link between work-related stress and musculoskeletal disorders [15].

In Italy, in the case of pathologies due to work-related stress, in order for Inail to deliver the relative economic services, the worker must demonstrate that the pathology is caused by an adverse working condition, reconstructing (through documentary and possibly testimonial evidence) work environment that contributed to the emergence of occupational stress disease.

Mental disorders can be considered of professional origin, and therefore eligible for compensation by Inail as an occupational disease, only if they are caused, even if only predominantly, by situations of organizational coercion, that is, if they involve clear and relevant consequences on the working position and on the possibilities of carrying out the work. Stress itself is not a disease, but its consequences may be. Continuous exposure to situations and sources of stress can in fact lead to physical and psychological somatization of the problem. In recent years, the evolution of pathologies and the data of occupational diseases in Italy reported by Inail makes evident the presence and growth of the phenomenon of work-related stress.

According to the European Agreement on work-related stress of 2004, stress is "a condition that can be accompanied by disorders or dysfunctions of a physical, psychological or social nature and is a consequence of the fact that some individuals do not feel able to meet the demands or to the expectations placed in them" [16]. Work-related stress can therefore potentially affect every workplace and every worker as it is caused by different aspects closely related to the organization and the work environment.

In Italy, the current regulatory framework, consisting of Legislative Decree 81/2008 and related laws, obliges employers to assess and manage the work-related stress risk on a par with all other risks, in acknowledgment of the contents of the European agreement. In this regard, the Permanent Advisory Commission for Occupational Health and Safety has developed the necessary information for assessing the risk of work-related stress, identifying a methodological path that represents the minimum level of implementation of the obligation. The Department of Medicine, Epidemiology, Occupational Hygiene, and the Environment has developed a Methodology for assessing and managing work-related stress risk and published a specific online platform that can be used by Italian companies to carry out risk assessment pursuant to Legislative Decree 81/2008.

The proposed method offers companies validated tools and specific resources, which can be used by companies following a sustainable and integrated approach, divided into phases, which involve the involvement of prevention figures and workers. The aspect of the risk from work-related stress, also in the assessment of the allowances recognized by Inail, which represent only the most evident and emerged aspect of a much broader phenomenon, show how the evolution of work and its organization, despite the perspective of Fourth Capitalism, it continues to produce conditions of risk to health and safety, whether physical, mental or psychological. In this dimension, the aspects connected to the digitization and its impact on working conditions must also be considered, which the spread of smart working during the months of the pandemic has made it particularly widespread everywhere, even in Italy.

7. The covid risk and the impact of the digitalization of work

The pandemic had a significant impact on every dimension of the world of work, but the one that was most disrupted was health and safety. The explosion of an event with disruptive potential in terms of risks to the health of workers and the entire population has led, in the space of a few days, to drastic choices with the closure of many activities and to stringent measures that have seen a vast adjustment by part of the companies. These have been committed, both from an organizational and economic point of view, not only to guarantee the minimum prevention measures (from sanitization to the distribution of masks, as many as 98% of Italian companies have done so) [17], but also to provide adequate information to employees (94.7%), provide specific training (90.4%), rotate staff or program staggered access and exits (70%), make various types of tests available to collaborators (52%) and exempt the most fragile workers or with specific assistance problems from the obligation to be present (46.2%). Measures that have transversally affected the business world, from large to small which, despite a 1000 difficulties, have nevertheless adapted their organizational and management models to the standards imposed by the pandemic: standards in many cases onerous, both from an organizational point of view than cheap. The efforts were rewarded by the results, with containment of accidents from Covid in the workplace and causes of mortality: as of March 31, 2021, Inail accounted for 165,000 accident reports from Covid, mostly concentrated in the health sector (67.5%), of which 551 with fatal outcome. This is a high figure, considering the overall impact of Covid accidents on the total of those reported (infections caused by the Sars-Cov-2 virus in 2020 accounted for 23.6% of reports and 33.3% of those fatal), but relatively contained when compared to the effects, in terms of infections and mortality, produced by the epidemic.

At the same time, the widespread use of agile work as the main tool for preventing the spread of infections in the workplace, in addition to containing the risk, has had the positive effect of producing a significant drop in accidents while traveling. This dynamic marks an important discontinuity with respect to the trends of recent years which, in the face of stability of accidents in the workplace, had seen the number of those in transit progressively increase, especially among women.

The development of smart working as a new organizational model, if on the one hand has positive effects with reference to accidents and mortality at work, on the other, poses new challenges in terms of health and safety. A growing responsibility of the worker is necessary and required, who are asked to collaborate to better organize their domestic work station, in order to ensure adequate safety and prevent the occurrence of accidents or the onset of diseases. In this context, the risk margins potentially linked to the safety of a work environment that can vary over time widen (27% of agile workers worked from a place other than their home, even for prolonged periods), which is not said it complies with the minimum plant safety regulations (electrical, fire prevention) or that it has adequate and equipped workplaces and environments according to ergonomic criteria.

To these aspects is added the risk of increased stress produced by the expansion of working times, by performance anxiety, by the weakening of company relations, and by the fear of marginalization, already identified by various surveys by almost half of the agile workers such as elements of the discomfort of working remotely. These are the first elements of an experience that is still being evaluated, but whose impact on the health and safety dimension could be disruptive, both in terms of limiting the accident phenomenon and innovating the prevention and safety logic, which must be made more functional to the new organizational models. The emergency, in addition to making "the risk" tangible and real, has brought this dimension to the center of the strategies and of the company organization, paving the way for an unexpected coincidence of interests between the parties: health protection on the one hand, and safeguarding business activity on the other. An important step which, induced by the emergency of the moment and the need to adopt all the necessary measures to contain risks and infections, also resulted in the launch of a more participatory model of health and safety management in the company, which has become a shared value between all the parties, who have undertaken to implement, in a logic of prevalent collaboration, the most suitable measures to protect the health of workers on the one hand and the business activity on the other. The extraordinary survey carried out by Istat in December 2020 [17] on Italian companies with more than three employees, clearly highlights from this point of view the significant effort made by Italian companies to adapt to health protocols and the new rules and obligations imposed by the pandemic. It should be considered that 58.7% of the companies had to make changes to the work environments to ensure spacing, through the use of barriers, signs to trace different paths: a measure that is strongly conditioned by the size of the structures, affecting especially the large ones with more than 250 employees, where "structural" interventions were made by 85.9% and to a lesser extent, but still important, the small ones, as even among companies with less than 10 employees, are 57% are involved in these types of initiatives. In the face of the measures relating to the work environment, the companies had to make important organizational interventions to ensure safety within the premises, in compliance with the health protocols provided. The experience of the last year has led to new leadership of companies and employees in the management of safety at work, which could mark an important step towards a more participatory and shared intervention logic.

The challenge of the Fourth Capitalism, the ongoing digitization, and the characteristics of the new organizational models of work entail in any case new risk factors for the health of citizens, which must be faced with tools, rules, and with a different culture of prevention, of work, and corporate well-being.

8. International health security and coordination of action to combat the accident phenomenon

What is dealt with in Italy by the institutions responsible for preventing and combating the phenomenon of accidents at work finds an international reference at the institutional level, first of all in the role of the International Labor Organisation (ILO), the World Labor Organization.

Worldwide, it is estimated that every 15 sec a worker dies on the job due to an accident at work or an occupational disease. Every 15 sec, 153 workers have an accident at work. It is also estimated that 6300 people die every day from work-related accidents or occupational diseases, causing more than 2.3 million deaths a year. The injuries which are prolonged work on-site annually 317 million, many of which involve sick leave from work. The human cost of these tragedies is enormous and the economic burden of inadequate occupational safety practices is estimated to be 4% of the world's gross domestic product each year.

The work that the ILO carries out in the field of health and safety at work intends to develop and increase awareness, worldwide, of the consequences of accidents, injuries, and occupational diseases in the workplace, through information and assistance activities for all male and female workers internationally, and supporting practical action at all levels. The ILO has adopted more than 40 conventions and recommendations relating specifically to occupational health and safety and has adopted over 40 codes of conduct. The recommendations and indications of the ILO constitute an important reference for the action of governments and in particular the Italian government, in its law enforcement policies, has carefully followed the various ILO indications, in particular in recent months on aspects relating to the return to the work safely during the Covid-19 pandemic. In particular, the ILO document of May 2020 [18], which defines the actions necessary for returning to work in safe conditions, should be mentioned. This tool provides guidance to employers, workers, and their representatives on preventive measures for a safe return to work in the context of Covid-19. The tool follows the ILO's established principles and methods on risk management for occupational safety and health and requires the involvement of workers. The tool must be adapted to national guidelines and does not address higher risk sectors, such as health services, and has been considered in the provisions adopted by the Italian government in recent months.

The European reference institution is the European Agency for Safety and Health at Work Occupational Safaty and Health Administration (EU-OSHA). This institution works to make EU workplaces safer, healthier, and more productive, for the benefit of companies, workers, and governments, and to foster a culture of risk prevention aimed at improving working conditions in Europe. In particular, these EU-OSHA benchmark actions need to be considered:

- Healthy and Safe Workplace campaigns: these biennial campaigns raise awareness of occupational health and safety (OSH) issues in Europe;

- The online interactive risk assessment (OiRA) project, which provides online tools for small and medium-sized enterprises to assess and manage risks in the workplace;

- The European Survey Of Entreprises On New And Emerging Risks (ESENER) survey: this comprehensive survey offers an instant description of how to manage health and safety risks in European workplaces;

- Forecasting projects: which highlight new and emerging OSH risks with specific forecasting projects.

The institutions that operate in Italy for prevention and safety at work act using the instrumentation and analysis carried out by the European OSHA Agency. In recent months, EU-OSHA is implementing a series of forecasting projects aimed at assessing the possible effects of new technologies and new ways of working as well as social changes on the health and safety of workers. Projects aim not only to identify new risks as they emerge but also to anticipate changes that could affect health and safety in the workplace. EU-OSHA foresight projects use a variety of methods, including literature reviews, expert consultations, and scenario development.

The purpose of this work program is to inform policymakers and to help define priorities for action and research. Foresight studies can have a major impact on decisions to be made, for example by helping policymakers find innovative solutions and promoting a long-term strategic approach.

The reference European policies and the indications of the European Commission must then be considered, which constitute the priority area of international health security for Italy. In this sense, the provisions of the EU Strategic Framework on health and safety in the workplace 2021–2027 must be considered: "Safety and health at work in a changing world of work" [19]. EU legislation on health and safety at work (OSH) is essential to protect the health and safety of the nearly 170 million workers in the EU. Protecting people from risks to health and safety in the workplace is in fact a key element in guaranteeing decent and lasting working conditions for all workers. This has made it possible to reduce occupational health risks and improve OSH standards within the EU and across all sectors.

However, challenges remain, and the covid-19 pandemic has exacerbated the risks that need to be addressed. The protection of the health and safety of workers, enshrined in the Treaties and the Charter of Fundamental Rights, is one of the basic elements of an EU economy serving citizens. The right to a safe and healthy workplace is reflected in Principle 10 of the European Pillar of Social Rights and is fundamental to achieving the United Nations Sustainable Development Goals, as well as being a constituent element of the European Union of health in progress of development.

The new OSHA 2021–2027 framework, announced in the European Pillar of Social Rights Action Plan, sets out the priorities and key actions needed to improve the health and safety of workers over the next few years in the post-world context pandemic, characterized by green and digital transitions, economic and demographic challenges, and the evolution of the concept of the traditional work environment.

9. Conclusions

Undoubtedly, smart working has had a very positive effect in terms of contraction of the accident phenomenon, allowing an important reduction of accidents during the journey that have always presented greater criticalities both in terms of management and prevention, also because they are not immediately related to the working environment. However, the evolution towards an agile work model, made up of growing hybridization between face-to-face and remote activities, also poses new challenges in terms of managing the health and safety of workers. Beyond the indications of the law, and the employers' provisions, it is evident that some typical elements of smart working, of remote work, as it has taken shape in the experience of the last year, raise many questions about the actual capacity for the protection of the health and safety of workers, where, beyond the training and training obligations of the employer, a large part of the responsibility is entrusted to the worker: think of the necessary electrical and fire safety to be guaranteed inside the elected home workplace, at the workstation, which must be defined and equipped according to ergonomic criteria or the possibility of carrying out work remotely from places and contexts other than the usual, for which it is difficult to imagine that conditions and safety procedures.

Mobility from one workplace to another, outside the company, represents a potential factor in increasing health risks. The alternation of places increases the risk of the inadequacy of domestic workstations, which already appears to be a "critical" factor for the health of workers. A survey carried out by the Labor Consultants Studies Foundation shows that in Italy [20], in May 2021, almost half of the employed working from home (48.3%, estimated at 2.6 million employees) complained of the onset of problems physical resulting from this aspect; an element that is particularly accentuated among men (50.4%) and among young people, where 53.6% report this type of problem. This is a fact attributable to the presumed less attention in compliance with procedures and precautions aimed at protecting health, which grows in contrast with advancing age, but also to the more frequent movement to workplaces other than one's home, which presumably present greater limits in terms of safety and suitability of the workstations.

Another aspect worthy of attention, for the implications in terms of health and well-being of the worker, is the increase in work stress, generated by the dilation of time, by performance anxiety, by the weakening of company relations, all aspects highlighted by the survey cited as a direct consequence of the use of agile work and which together can contribute to causing an increase in work-related stress and particular pathologies connected to it. According to this survey, almost half of smart working workers complain of greater stress and performance anxiety. Even the distortion of relationships with colleagues, bosses, customers, based on physical distancing, in the long-run has counterproductive effects for about one worker out of two: 49.7% in fact report the worsening of the climate in the company, the weakening of working relationships; 47% feel marginalized with respect to the dynamics of organizations, while about 40% begin to report real disaffection towards work. Finally, about a third (33%) declare that remote work is penalizing their career and professional growth.

The digitization of the way the work is carried out must therefore be considered for what it really is: it is not the mere introduction of new technical and organizational tools, but the promotion of a real context, a different environment that determines an overall impact on conditions of work and can lead to opportunities and problems at the same time. In general, the analysis of the trend in these months of progressive exit from the pandemic of accidents at work, occupational diseases, and the impact of smart working and work stress confirms that in this historical phase it is very important to avoid changes in the work induced by the economy compromise the conditions of well-being, human relations, and the reconciliation between lifetimes and work times. The challenge of well-being at work is the factor that goes with a decrease in the risk of accidents and illnesses. This is true in Italy as in the rest of Europe.

Author details

Romano Benini
Sociology of Welfare, Link Campus University, Rome, Italy

*Address all correspondence to: r.benini@unilink.it

IntechOpen

References

[1] Decreto legislativo. n. 81 del Testo unico per la sicurezza sul lavoro [Consolidated text for workplace safety]. 2008

[2] Bollettino trimestrale Inail terzo trimestre. [Quarterly bulletin Inail]. 2021

[3] Bollettino trimestrale Inail secondo trimestre. [Quarterly bulletin Inail]. 2021

[4] Rapporto nazionale Inail [National Report Inail]. 2020

[5] Rapporto nazionale Inail [National Report Inail]. 2019

[6] Rapporto nazionale Inail [National Report Inail]. 2018

[7] Rapporto nazionale Inail [National Report Inail]. 2017

[8] Sennett R. The Corrosion of Character, The Personal Consequences Of in the New Capitalism. New York-London: Norton; 1998. [Trad. it. L'uomo flessibile. Le conseguenze del nuovo capitalismo sulla vita personale. Milano: Feltrinelli; 1999]

[9] Topol E. Deep Medicine: How Artificial Intelligence Can Make Healthcare Human Again. New York: Basic Books; 2019

[10] Eherenberg R. The Uneasy society. Paris: Odile Jacob; 2010 [trad. italiana *La società del disagio. Il mentale ed il sociale*. Torino: Einaudi]

[11] Rapporto nazionale Inail [National Report Inail]. 2015

[12] Rapporto nazionale Inail [National Report Inail]. 2016

[13] Rapporto nazionale Inail [National Report Inail]. 2017

[14] Analisi 2021 dell'Osservatorio indipendente di Bologna morti sul lavoro [Independent Observatory of Bologna on the fallen from work]. 2021

[15] EU-OSHA—European Agency for Safety and Health at Work. Expert Forecast on Emerging Psychosocial Risks Related to Occupational Safety and Health. Luxembourg: Office for Official Publications of the European Communities; 2007

[16] Implementation of the European autonomous framework Agreement on work-related stress. Report by the European Social Partners Adopted at the Social Dialogue Committee on 18 June 2008

[17] Report su "Situazione e prospettive delle imprese nell'emergenza sanitaria Covid-19". Published respectively on 15 June: https://www.istat.it/it/archivio/244378; and on 14 December 2020: https://www.istat.it/it/archivio/251618

[18] ILO Standards and Covid 19. 2020. Available from: https://www.ilo.org/global/topics/coronavirus/impacts-andresponses/lang--en/index.htm

[19] EU Commission. Report: "Safety and Health at Work in a Changing World of Work". Available from: https://ec.europa.eu/ social/main.jsp?catId=148

[20] Report 'Gli italiani e il lavoro dopo la grande emergenza. Fondazione studi Consulenti del lavoro [Italians and work after the great emergency. Foundation for labor consultant studies]

www.ingramcontent.com/pod-product-compliance
Lightning Source LLC
Chambersburg PA
CBHW081559190326
41458CB00015B/5653